Behind My

Bethany and Julie Simpson

Review:
An insight into lives of the child and family coping with the devastating disease Juvenile Arthritis. A must read for parents and medical staff alike who look after children with a chronic illness.

Children's Community Nursing Team

Bethany & Julie Simpson © Copyright 2008

All characters are fictional and any resemblance to persons alive or dead
is entirely coincidental

All rights reserved

No parts of this publication may be reproduced, stored in a retrieval system,
or transmitted in any form or by any means, electronic, mechanical,
photocopying, recording or otherwise without the prior permission of the
copyright owner.

British Library Cataloguing In Publication Data
A Record of this Publication is available
from the British Library

ISBN 978-1-84685-891-8

First Published 2008 by
Exposure Publishing,
an imprint of
Diggory Press Ltd
Three Rivers, Minions, Liskeard, Cornwall, PL14 5LE, UK
and of Diggory Press, Inc.,
Goodyear, Arizona, 85338, USA
WWW.DIGGORYPRESS.COM

Acknowledgements from Bethany:

To my friends, you know who you are.

To Dr Armon, Kit and Judy, Suzanne and her team

To the teachers at my school, especially Mrs. K

Acknowledgments from Julie:

To Karen, who without your encouragement this book would still be on my computer. Thanks also to Jo and Suzanne

To Steve and Debbie for your honest advice

To Vicki, you have helped to improve Bethany's future.

To Sue, Debbie, Alison, and Sam for all your care and support

To our family and friends for all your support even though I know there were times you did not know how to help.

To Suzanne and the therapy team at the Newberry Clinic, you are truly special people.

To Dr. Wyllie, thank you for being such a good listener and the staff at the Falkland Surgery.

To the staff at Bethany's school who probably do not know how much they have helped her feel secure enough to learn I am so grateful

To Dr Kate Armon, to Kit and Judy for helping give my child back her childhood.

To Carol our Homeopath, without your remedies things would have been very bleak.

To the Bradwell 2nd Brownies, thank you for the purple evening and for including Bethany at all times.

To my friends and work colleagues who have listened.

To Norma for teaching her to love play the piano.

To Barry and John at Hot Springs, Highways Nurseries.

Behind My Smile

Bethany and *Julie Simpson*

CONTENTS

Bethany's Journey   *9-53*

Julie's Journey   *55-106*

Bethany's Journey:

CHAPTER ONE

What's happening to me!

I think all stories start at the beginning, however I cannot remember the beginning of my story. I have heard a lot about when I was two and had a sore knee, and they called it childhood Arthritis. That doesn't mean much to me now but I can remember the last two years single second of them

It all started for me just the same as usual. I went as usual. I was in year three. I had a lovely teacher and some great close friends, with one special friend. Everything seemed the same; assembly, work not to bad, though my writing had seemed to have got bigger and scribblier, oh well the teacher hadn't said anything maybe I was imagining it, it's wasn't too bad. Funny though something else did not feel right, I felt a bit stiff. It was break next, so I finished my worksheet.

We went out to play as we always do, had a run around, and played some games I forgot to mention that the week before my friend Anna accidentally fell on top of me when she fell off the bench. I went down on my knees it was sore but I just got up and carried on I didn't like to make a fuss.

Anyway where was I oh that's right playtime my legs felt strange. I didn't seem to be getting very far and I couldn't bend my knee. I didn't say anything. Oh no just my luck, it was mum watching me from the school nursery window. I didn't mind her working here. I wish she wouldn't keep spying on me. There she was still watching. I was standing still and I was not going to let her see me, she would not get off my back, she has a beady eye that just doesn't miss anything. Anyway I would be fine when I get home, I'm sure I would be back to normal.

No such luck as soon as we got home the questions started. 'Is your leg sore Bethany you seemed to be dragging it today lets have a look.' Oh great here we go, I was hoping to go and play with my friend tonight.

Then the panic on her face started and she wanted to look all over me, she looked at my hands and gasped. I started crying and ran to my bedroom. My little sister came up 'Go away leave me alone' I screamed at her. Just then Dad came up 'lets have a look poppet, mum says your legs and fingers are stiff can I see'. I showed him and again the same panic on his face. He went downstairs; it was that moment my life changed beyond belief.

CHAPTER TWO

My eighth birthday

Mum and Dad took me to see the GP who confirmed it looked like the Juvenile Arthritis had recurred and he was going to write off to the hospital. It was my birthday two days later and mum had arranged a party well two parties the first one for my sister Mariella who was four and for me. I would be eight.

It was held at Smart Kids, a centre for Autistic children. It had a huge trampoline, ball pit, bouncy castle and a cool outside area with a sandpit, slides, trikes and climbing frames. I had a nice time, kept a smile on my face but to tell the truth, this is my downfall apparently. I don't tell the truth too much - well it seems to upset everyone so much, so I prefer not to say anything at all that might upset anyone.

I did feel sore and stiff and my left leg didn't seem to keep up with my other leg. I found it hard to climb and to bend and had to sit on a chair to have the party food. Great all the others were sat on the floor and there was I sitting on a chair like the odd one out. I hate, hate, and hate being the odd one out; I just want to be the same as everyone else. People kept staring at me, well the grown ups anyway. I couldn't enjoy the party because of my silly stiff leg; my sister had a lovely time at her half of the party.

Mum and Dad had bought me a bike for my birthday but guess what I couldn't ride it. Dad took it back to the shop, the man adapted it for me, and Dad changed the brakes, as I couldn't squeeze them. I found it easier to ride the bike than I did to walk. I didn't feel so different when I was riding the bike, I didn't feel like the odd one out.

CHAPTER THREE

The first hospital appointment

Mum and Dad took me to the local hospital to see the same doctor who treated me when I was two apparently. I was so frightened, I was taken into a small room and weighed and measured. We were then shown into another room with, well, it looked like hundreds of grown ups in white coats. I'm sure that there wasn't hundreds. However, that's how it seemed to me. I didn't understand what he was saying, I had stopped listening and gone into a world of my own however, looking at mum and dad's faces it wasn't good news that was for sure. He did say something about making me better but he also talked about blood tests, it all sounded horrible.

I met Suzanne who was going to become quite well known to me in the future. She was my Physiotherapist and she was the one who gave me lots of exercises to do and came in the water with us at the hydrotherapy pool. I was very scared and kept going over the same thing in my head 'why can't they leave me alone'.

Everything really changed after that; all they talked about was Arthritis. Mum and Dad walked about with a sad look on their faces. Do you know I still can't say that I have Arthritis I can't do it. I suppose that would make it too real. Mum and Dad stopped talking about my illness when I was around as I got very distressed and really couldn't cope with it. I used to find them whispering and I used to make sure Mum couldn't speak to anyone on the phone in case it was about me. Even when it wasn't about me, I caused a scene and mum kept saying that I was putting her in a very difficult situation. I didn't care and I just wanted her to stop talking about me – FULL STOP.

CHAPTER FOUR

Carried like a baby

We went to visit my new school just down the road. We went to see where we would be going in September it was June now and I had no idea at that time that I would be taking my Arthritis with me to that school and still have it two years later. I am glad I did not know how bad things were going to get for me.

Something really awful happened during that visit, my legs wouldn't work, my lovely teacher saw this and she carried me back to school, in front of all the class. Can you imagine how I felt 8 years old and being carried like a baby?

I got a few strange looks that day. When I got home mum knew as my lovely teacher had told her. Mum looked confused not as confused as I am. I didn't want to talk to anyone when we got back to school, I feel so STUPID, STUPID, STUPID.

I was finding it hard to write and my writing was very big. Mum looked back at my old school books and was very upset as my writing had been bad before and they hadn't noticed. I think Mum and Dad thought it was their fault but I felt like it was my fault as before all this had happened, things were okay and now they were HORRIBLE.

CHAPTER FIVE

My new life – It sucks

I was taking all this horrible medicine and had to go to Hydrotherapy and do many exercises at home too. Great - when could I just play then?

I did like Hydrotherapy though, my physiotherapist Suzanne was really nice, the water was lovely, and warm I couldn't feel the pain so much.

I wish I could live in a pool – we played games in the water after we had done the exercises. I could swim. I had lessons but now it was hard to lift my shoulders much and I was finding it hard to grip onto the side of the pool.

The other children didn't seem to feel the same as me. They didn't seem to mind when their mum talked to Suzanne about their symptoms. I hated it and caused such a fuss that mum didn't even like to answer Suzanne's questions, as I got soooo mad.

There was another lady who helped with the games. . She was nice and made us laugh. I did well in the games in the pool, I was the oldest in the group, and it felt good to do well.

I didn't do games or PE at school so I felt almost okay at the Hydrotherapy sessions. I went back to school after Hydrotherapy. Mum always gave me something to eat in the car, as I was very hungry. I missed Drama on the Friday morning; I loved Drama too, so I felt a bit sad.

Most of the time I felt low, I had to have everything done for me, as my hands were so USELESS, I wished that I could disappear. I wished, I wished, oh what was the point, wishes don't come true anyway. I was stuck in a body that didn't work; I needed help to climb the stairs. I had to be lifted in and out of the bath and the toothpaste tube was squeezed for me. Oh, I could go on and on, it's a long list and I just wanted to be as I was before, like all the other children. Why me, why was this happening to me

I know Mum and Dad were so worried so I tried not telling them about the pain. I couldn't really write very much and I didn't finish the QCA tests at school so I had to go to my new school with no results. Great wasn't it.

CHAPTER SIX

Centre Parcs – Eight and in a buggy

We were going to Centre Parcs the next weekend and I was really looking forward to it.

Our villa was quite a walk. Walk - that's what I used to do. My legs seemed to have forgotten how to walk. It was so embarrassing Mum and Dad had to go and ask for a buggy for me. They only had a double buggy so Mariella sat in the back and I went in the front. It was really horrible as children kept staring and grown ups too. I was so angry with them that I stuck my tongue out at them. I just wanted to disappear so no one could see me.

When we got home, I got very sore and stiff and found everything difficult. Dad had to lift me out of bed and they had to carry me around. I couldn't flush the toilet anymore; I couldn't bend to get in and out of bed or the bath. I couldn't do much at all really and I felt really stupid. I sat on a chair at school now – one that meant I could reach the floor with the feet, there was a bit of confusion at school really, I think they didn't know how much I couldn't do anymore.

I could barely hold my dinner tray. Mum really embarrassed me as I was waiting for the dinner lady to take my tray but mum took it out of my hands and I ended up having packed lunches. This did work out better as my friend opened all my packets for me as I was finding it hard to lift and carry things but I wasn't going to tell them that. I feel really cross with Mum now, she won't stop fussing. I needed help to do everything I had to give up my recorder as the music teacher said my fingers kept seizing up.

CHAPTER SEVEN

The worst summer

The summer holidays came and it wasn't like any other summer holiday I had had before. Things seemed very sad, a buggy arrived for me, a huge one and I hated it

The holidays were horrid; it felt like everyone was mean to me. A couple of girls kept coming round pretending to want to play with me and then braiding their hair with my new hair beads and running home. Mum wasn't happy; I couldn't even get on the floor to tidy up the mess they had made. I wanted to scream, shout and kick out, and I did all this and it just made mum cry.

The girls did not live around here, and mum hoped they would get fed up, and move onto someone else. They did eventually and I tried to mix in with the other children, but I felt so useless.

Mum and Dad said that they would buy us a guinea pig to try to cheer us up. Nanny and Grandad came over to look after us while they went up to Cromer. We were excited when they came home. When we had a close look at the little bundle wrapped up in a blanket we realised that it was a puppy. We called her Honey and we had lots of fun with her. She did take my mind off all the horrid stuff, for a while but she did nibble my fingers and they were sore. Mum was sad about this and kept saying things weren't meant to be like this.

I loved being with my best friend she was great. I didn't have to say anything to her; she opened doors for me and made things much easier. I could hide my hands, I put them behind my back I hated them – the doctor called them SPINDLY, He didn't care how I felt when he said that. I was smiling all the time now, as people seem happy when I smile.

CHAPTER EIGHT

Methotrexate

We went back to the hospital; the doctor was talking a lot, and looking at me. I hated it so much that I gave Mum horrible looks. She was getting tearful then but I couldn't help it I didn't want to make her cry but I felt that it was her fault for telling them. Dad took me out of the room Dad; I hated it when they are talking about me.

That week I had to take some new medicine. I couldn't manage to swallow it, so a nurse came. I tried again to swallow it, but I just couldn't. The nurses were not allowed to touch the tablets nor were Mum and Dad. I was crying and mum was very upset too. It was so unfair.

The nurse arrived a few days later saying I had to have an injection. I started screaming and lashing out just as I did when I had the blood tests.

When it was over everyone made such a fuss of me and I ran up to my bedroom. Mum said that this would make me feel better and help me. I hated that nurse I never wanted to see her again.

Actually, I did learn to like her quite a lot in the following weeks. The nurses came in once a week to give me my injection and they turned out to be very nice.

CHAPTER NINE

Splints, sweats and night terrors

I didn't feel right I was crying and screaming- mostly at mum, it was horrible really horrible and I kept having horrible dreams. Mum said that I was awake when I had them.

Oh I haven't told you that I had to wear splints on my legs at night, my legs aren't straight and if I didn't wear them, my leg was stuck in the morning and I couldn't get it down.

When I had them made at the hospital, my dad came with me. He said that I screamed like a banshee. I have no idea what a banshee is but she must have a loud scream. It was so hot and it hurt, there is no way I thought I was going to wear them. However, like everything else in those days, how I feel didn't count anymore.

Have you ever tried to sleep with hard itchy plaster Paris legs? It was horrid. Mum and Dad came in to help me fix them on and off in the night. I couldn't get through the whole night, no way. Mum had to prop the covers up as my ankles hurt when the sheets pressed down on them.

Everything changed in my life we couldn't do anything any more, no walks, no parks, no play areas.

I could sit on my swing in the garden. However, I couldn't swing it because I couldn't grip the rope and have to keep myself on with my elbows. I also had to be careful not to be knocked into as my joints especially my fingers hurt. I stood back from everyone, as was frightened to be knocked over again, that's how it all started in the first place.

I stayed in a break times with my friend and kept away from busy areas as best I could. My chair had a wooden bit on it so that I couldn't put my feet on it, it was strange at first, but I'm okay with it now, I was very, very tired now and weepy.

CHAPTER TEN

The power of music

Mum asked me if I wanted to learn to play the piano, my cousin had been learning, I think mum thought it would make me feel a bit better. Well she was right.

My teacher was lovely and I enjoyed learning the notes it wasn't easy for me to play but I found it helpful.

Mum and Dad bought me a second hand piano and it went in my bedroom. When I was finding the pain too much I played and it made me feel better. If I was low I thumped the keys, I wasn't screaming as much now I had the piano and it did help me when I want to kick out and scream – it made me feel a bit calmer.

Twinkle twinkle little star

How I wonder what you are?

Up above the world so high

Like a diamond in the sky

Twinkle twinkle little star

How I wonder what you are?

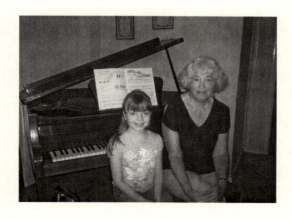

CHAPTER ELEVEN

No one knew how I felt

They started to fuss over me now. I felt stupid. Mum had to tell Brown Owl that I was not well. I love Brownies though so I am happy that I could still go. I tried to join in, but it' was hard to join in the games but I had a go. I didn't mind sitting on a chair at school so much but I do wish I could be the same as the others. I hated it when at PE and games, it looked fun but I couldn't do it.

I was meeting other children with my illness but no one my age. I could see the other children are sore by the way they were moving. I tried harder to hide my pain and I kept smiling.

Mum tried to find someone that has the same illness as me, more my age hoping that, I will talk to her. I said that would be good but she couldn't find anyone. The only girl we found on the through the Contact a Friend lived in New Zealand. She couldn't be further away, just my luck.

Every morning I had to wake up not knowing which bit of me is going to hurt the most. The mornings are bad as I am very stiff and have to go down the stairs sideways. It takes ages and mum had to help me get dressed.

Dad had changed our taps so I can use them. I can't even open a packet of crisps without someone helping me. Nothing is the same anymore; even my little sister can do more than me. I can't bend my knees. They don't think that I will ever be able to bend my legs again.

CHAPTER TWELVE

My hairs falling out

Something really, really horrible happened then. It was my hair, my lovely long thick blond hair. It started to come out when I combed it. I was so upset I went to tell mum. I know it was very early and mum was still in bed. I was crying and showing mum all the hair. She looked strange. I had never seen her look strange that strange before. She seemed to pull herself together, but she and dad had a row and I went back to my bedroom. It's all my fault mum and dad were always arguing. I just wanted everything to go back to normal, would it ever go back to normal?

Mum was not going to work she was very tearful I knew that she was trying to put on a brave face but its hard to do that all the time. Mum showed me a website of things children who have my problems had written. It was sad and we both cried. I felt like those children. They had drawn pictures describing their pain. It was really horrible mum kept crying and asked if I felt like that. I ran to my bedroom.

Twinkle twinkle little star

How I wonder what you are

up above the sky so high

Like a diamond in the sky

Twinkle twinkle little star

How I wonder what you are.

CHAPTER THIRTEEN

Christmas and New Year

They were calling me disabled. I am so angry so angry and I was shouting at mum all the time. Christmas came and we got lots of pressies.

I got Ninetendo with dogs; we seem to be getting more presents now. We had lots of people round and things were good. We went to my Nanny and Grandad's for Christmas Day. It was lovely, everyone seemed happy again and I wished that day could have lasted forever. Wishes don't come true though.

After Christmas, we went back to the hospital and mum told the Doctor that the medicine for my tummy was upsetting me. I was taking it to protect my tummy against the anti-inflammatory. He told me that I didn't need the anti-inflammatory any more as the methotrexate was working well.

Well mum followed the Doctor's advice. The school stopped giving me lunchtime doses. However, I got a bit stiff and then very stiff and sore and couldn't do much. I was hobbling around, this was even worse than before.

When the nurse came to inject my methotrexate, mum told her that my joint's were hot and swollen. When the nurse looked at me, I walked sideways. I was trying to hide it again, and I felt so stupid. In the end I started back on the anti-inflammatory medicine again, it was all very confusing.

I went to the medical room at school to have the medicine. I also went in first to dinner with a friend and had to use special knives and forks. I used my fingers at home; as it was easier, otherwise it took such a long time to eat. I didn't like a lot of the food that I used to like anymore. My stomach was playing me up again.

We went to see the physiotherapist lots of times I liked her she made me feel nice but she kept giving me lots of exercises to do. It took ages and ages. I had bands, bouncers and balls; it's not fair I was really cross and angry. I had to have my eyes checked as well as the Arthritis could get into my eyes; it's was like an evil monster crawling around my body.

Mum kept making lots of phone calls and its really upsetting me now as she's whispering a lot. Why does she keep talking about me. My injections take longer now, as there is more medicine in it. It stings so much and a get a bruise afterwards. My hair looks scruffy all the time and darker and I feel sick and I am gagging a lot. I can't eat very much and everyone keeps saying how thin and pale I am – great.

CHAPTER FOURTEEN

The Piano Festival

In March, my piano teacher asked me if I would like to play in a Piano Festival. She said I could play Twinkle Twinkle Little Star and Old MacDonald Had a Farm.

I practiced on my piano at home. I enjoyed playing my piano. It is in my bedroom.

It was so funny when the piano arrived. The men had to bring in up to my bedroom. It's a mini piano made in the 1930's. It took them an hour. They had to slide it up on a piece of wood. They got so hot and bothered. Mum had to get them cold drinks so they could recover.

Going back to the Piano Festival, we arrived in time and sat with my teacher Norma. She is so lovely I really found it good to be with her. Norma didn't know too much about my illness and didn't even mention it. I really enjoyed going to see her. She gave me tests using smarties to remember the notes; I wish they did that sort of thing at school. Maybe everyone would remember their spellings if they got smarties as a reward.

I played my pieces and I wasn't too nervous. I think I did okay. After all the other children had finished, the examiner thanked everybody and then read out our results and a few things about our playing. I got a merit and he said:

Twinkle Twinkle Little Star - A steady, firm performance. Try now to achieve a bouncy acceato and look at the shapes.

Old MacDonald – This was a fluent performance. Try now to develop a compact hand position and curved fingers. Keep up the good work.

Mum and Dad were proud of me, however a little upset that the examiner had mentioned my hands, as I was not able to hold them that way.

When things got bad and I wouldn't speak to mum about how much pain I was in, she asked me to tell her about each joint on a scale of one to ten. Ten was the most pain. Sometimes I wouldn't even do this, I know I made things difficult but I just couldn't say it, I wanted it all to go away.

One day when I was not doing so well, I went up to play on my piano and thumped the keys. Mum asked to play the notes to show her how things were for me. I thumped the low keys and then she asked again for me to score the pain in each joint using the piano. I didn't mind doing this so we used the range of keys and I played each one to show the pain in each joint. Mum was over the moon that I was actually telling her but of course, I wasn't telling her because I can't tell her. We used the piano all the time from then on.

CHAPTER FIFTEEN

School and all that smiling

At school I kept smiling, the teachers asked if I'm all right and I smiled and nodded and they went away. My teacher was nice, he watched me a lot and sometimes rang mum to ask her things about me.

Something so horrid happened. I felt so stupid, we had to do our QCA's at school and mum told me that I would have a support worker to help me with the writing. I was so angry. I hid in the wardrobe and refused to go the school. Did they think I was dumb now. I was very upset and frightened but I wasn't going to tell let anyone know.

I told mum that I wanted to die, and to leave me alone. I hate to upset her but I had had enough.

Anyway, doing the tests was just as bad as it gets. I had a lady from the support centre to help me and I kept telling her what to write, well whispering it. She kept writing the wrong thing, so I snatched the pen out of her hand and did it myself. I bet everyone thought I had turned dumb as well as everything else as she helped children who need help with their work. I just needed help because my fingers ache and ache and ache.

I was having lots of medicines, some at school, some at home and that injection. I didn't mind the blood tests so much now as they don't take the blood from my hand anymore, that really hurt me and I couldn't stop screaming. Mum cried and cried so much sometimes that I don't think she could have any tears left.

My sister was getting on my nerves; she has started to act, as a little baby. She has decided she can't get dressed or do anything. Mum is very sad about that and I don't think she has a clue what to do. She mentioned it to one of my nurses when they came to give me my injection, and mum was told that it is very common for a little sister to be jealous. I found that weird, very weird, why would anyone be jealous of me. I move like an old lady not a child. She can run, play, and do everything. Does she want the injection and all the fuss? She's really getting me down.

CHAPTER SIXTEEN

Easter and the car crash

Mum had arranged for us to go and see her old school friend at Easter. Her daughter was thirteen and she had been mum and dad's bridesmaid at their wedding.

It was a long way so we were going to stay at a hotel and then see mum's sister and her grandchildren, well that would have been nice if things had gone to plan, but it did not.

The first bit was okay, we went to see mums friend. They have huge house it is three stories high, how did I manage to get to the top? – Well with great difficulty! We had lunch and then started to go to the hotel.

We were lost as usual and ended up on a huge roundabout. We were just about to take our turning and then a car hit us. The shock was too much for me, my shoulder hurt but I didn't say anything, it all got a bit out of hand. The woman who hit us was nasty and kept shouting she was frightening us. We managed to pull away after mum had called the police as the woman was acting very weirdly.

We got to the hotel, but as you can imagine it, was all upsetting and mum took me straight into the swimming pool to try to loosen me up a bit.

The next day we met my auntie, uncle and cousin at a farm but I couldn't walk at all. I was too upset to go in my buggy. We had a nice time and Dad carried me on his shoulders, as I was very light.

CHAPTER SEVENTTEN

Brownie Camp

Brownie camp was at a special needs school in Norwich. It had a Hydrotherapy pool and a Sensory chilling out room. Mum and Dad had spoken to Brown Owl and she said they would do my exercises with me and let me go in the pool everyday.

I couldn't stay the nights though as I had my splints to wear. In addition, I couldn't bend down to get on the beds that all the other girls were going to sleep on.

Mum, Dad and Mariella took me, we got lost. When we got there, all the beds were ready. I felt a bit sad to be the odd one out again, as I had a chair with my shoebox sitting on it. Our shoebox was to hold all the things that we would make; it was the theme of bugs. Mine was covered in ladybirds and butterflies.

I went home everyday and Dad and Mariella took me back in the mornings. We tucked into bacon sandwiches every morning when we arrived.

I really enjoyed it and was happy that I was able to join in. Brown Owl let me go in the hydrotherapy Pool every day and they had permission to help me get dressed as my fingers were very stiff and it was difficult. One of the older helpers wrote my diary out for me. I also did my physiotherapy at the camp.

These exercises made me ache and I hated doing them. Mum insisted that I had to build up some muscles and to try to keep my joints moving.

CHAPTER EIGHTEEN

My meltdown

I had started to feel worse and my knees were even more swollen. I felt strange and couldn't stop screaming. I was so sore and so tired I couldn't smile much. I saved my smiles for when someone asked me how I am. I then put on a great big smile and say fine. They seemed fine with that well everyone except mum and dad, as they are not so easily convinced.

I kept dropping things especially drinks so I had to use plastic cups. My fingers seemed to have forgotten how to grip. Mum was so worried about me; she got very sad and hardly smiled.

The next hospital appointment seemed different somehow. Karen, one of my nurses said she would come in with us. Mum said that she was going to ask me to see another doctor, one at another hospital. Great, great, great. It was all to do with mum going to a talk with her friend. She seemed even more strange than usual.

When we went in mum seemed to be quite cross and kept interrupting. She had a word with the doctor and she seemed pleased he was nodding. I could not tell you what they were saying as I switched off and went into my own world where things were not so horrid.

When we left mum and dad were pleased and kept smiling. I haven't seen them like that for a long time and dad keeps saying its so stressful and I know that its all my fault – it wasn't like this before it all started.

CHAPTER NINETEEN

My new hospital

A couple of weeks later mum and dad took me to another hospital to meet a new doctor she was called a Rheumotologist and I really didn't want to go. I just wanted to be left alone.

She showed us into a small room. The nurse came in. There was another lady, a physiotherapist. My knees were sore. I hobbled like a hundred year old to the room and sat on a chair. The doctor was a lady and she looked very kind. She asked many questions and examined me. She looked at me differently to all the others and seemed to see where it hurt the most. She was asking mum lots of questions. Mum started sobbing and asked her to help me. It was weird, but the doctor said she would help me. Do you think mum stopped sobbing then – no, she didn't. Oh then I was weighed and measured. How do you think it felt a nine year old to come out at a baby weight? That is what I weighed the same as a baby.

We spend all day with the Nurse, her name was Kit, and she was lovely. She talked about Brownies as she pushed me around in a wheelchair. I had to have blood tests and x-rays. Dad bought me some sandwiches, as I was very hungry.

When we went back to join the Doctor she said that she wanted me to stay in hospital and to go on a drip. I started to cry and kicked out; they were all trying to calm me down. Kit took me to the ward to show me where I would be staying for two nights; they said that Mum could stay too. It was too much for me and I refused to so the Doctor asked me if I would keep down some tablets instead. I agreed and she gave me eight tablets to take and said that she was going to change all my medicines. Mum had given me some homeopathy tissue salts to stop me crying.

Dad went and got the medicine from the hospital and we were asked to come back next week. When we drove home Mum and Dad were almost, dare I say, happy. I was so tired that I fell asleep.

CHAPTER TWENTY

The School Trip

We went to a wildlife park called Africa Alive for our school trip. Mum had to be one of the helpers as I was going to have to use my buggy. I was hoping that no one would say anything mean to me.

We were in groups and I had a little walk to start with but my legs weren't working and it hurt. I didn't say anything but mum told me to hop in. I gave mum one of those looks, I know that I upset her when I did it but I couldn't help it. I always took it out on mum.

We went around the park with one of my friend's mums and enjoyed looking at all the animals. We took a packed lunch with us and ate that, and then a lady showed us some snakes and talk about Africa.

Things were ok until we turned the corner. There was a boy about seven I suppose and he started pointing at me and laughing saying that I was to big to be in a baby's buggy.' just like that. Those words tore through me. I couldn't see anyone as my eyes were stinging with the tears and I felt so ANGRY. I had a bottle, a plastic bottle in my hand. I threw it with all my might. Mum tried to calm me down she gave me one of my homeopathic tissue salts, which make me feel a bit better. However, the day was ruined.

Mum was so angry and I really didn't know what she was going to do next. All my friends are cross with what he had said and I could not smile now. I really couldn't smile then. I want to scream, scream, cry, and just disappear into thin air.

35

It was a shame as mum got very down then. She had told me that no one would be unkind to me. I think she felt that she had let me down.

It took a long time for me to recover and began to talk again. When I had calmed down. Mum explained that he did not mean to hurt my feelings and he probably wished that he had kept his mouth shut.

Anyway, the buggy was changed for a wheelchair and I felt better in that. People still stared at me but I got used to it and as mum said, we can either sit at home and do nothing or go out and enjoy what we can do.

Mum was always telling me about other children that were unwell and has even offered to take me to meet some. I think she wants to show me that I am not the only one suffering and that some children are dying. We sent some money to the Starlight Wish Foundation and hoped that it would help a child have their wish.

CHAPTER TWENTY-ONE

More injections and play sessions

When we went back to the hospital the next week, the doctor and Kit were pleased that I looked a bit brighter. I was feeling well, not so stiff, and not so sore but I was very, very hungry. Mum said that she couldn't keep up with me. I was eating so much, had gained some weight and guess what, I wasn't a baby anymore. I weighed three stones; I had only been two stones and something before.

My nana had been saying how thin I was for a long time so maybe she would be happy now.

Mum had to work fewer mornings, as we had to go to the hospital twice a week. Mum and dad were being trained to give me the new injections. It felt like we were always there.

I met Judy, she was a play worker she spent some time with me, to help me feel a bit better. We made a folder about all the things that I like and that I am good at doing. Every time I had a blood test or injection, I could choose a sticker.

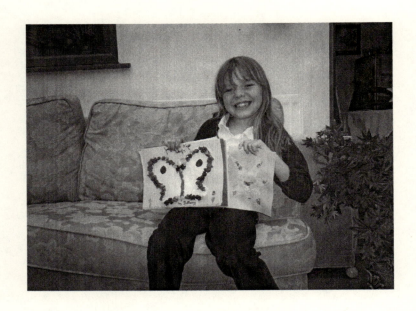

CHAPTER TWENTY-TWO

My Heart

When we first met my new doctor, she said that I had a heart murmur and that this would need to be checked out. This seemed to freak mum and dad out. They tried to tell me that it was nothing and that mum had had a murmur herself when she was young and she had grown out of it.

The day we had to go and have it checked out was not a nice day. My little sister had decided on this day of all days that she couldn't walk. My dad was very upset; as she was due to go to school whilst they took me to the hospital, which was over 20 miles away. Dad kept getting more and more in a panic and called mum. Mum was not having any of it and tricked Mariella into walking. It was all about

Mariella wanting attention because she knew I had to go to the hospital.

I think that was the worst stunt she has pulled yet, poor dad he was almost having a breakdown. Mum was not happy at all but felt so sorry for Mariella wondering what on earth was going around in her head to pretend that she couldn't walk. She must have been desperate if she wanted to be like me.

We took Mariella to school and then set off to the hospital. You will not believe this but half way to the hospital, mum gets a call on her mobile. She could see that it was Mariella's school and was told that Mariella needed to be sent home. Mum blurted out 'was it her legs' thinking that she must have pulled the wool over the teachers eyes, but she had a sticky eye. Mum had to ring my nanny and granddad and they went to collect her.

When we got to the hospital mum had gone to pieces. She was crying, and crying and said that she couldn't come in with me. This was strange for mum as she is always by my side so dad came in. I had a cold liquid put on my heart and she used a scanner. She told dad I had a small murmur and gave him a report to give to the doctor who we were going to see next. Mum was relieved that it wasn't bad news. I didn't really understand what was going on at all. The doctor was happy with the result and talked about my new injections.

CHAPTER TWENTY-THREE

Summer trips to the hospital - for my new injections

We had been given the date of 7 July 2006 to start the new injections. We had to go to Norwich twice a week on a Monday and Friday. Mum and dad had to learn how to do the injections. I wasn't looking forward to that and I didn't ever think that my dad would inject me.

I liked Kit the nurse. I was already used to having the Methotrexate injected in my thigh. Now I was going to have a methotrexate leg and an etanacept leg. We were told it was very important not to get them mixed up.

I always saw the play worker Judy and I enjoyed making the sticker charts, and loved taking the doll's blood test. We used a real needle and pulled out the red jam into the syringe, this was good fun. I also had turns in using the laptop and drew some pictures, which I saved.

We always went to the canteen and had sandwiches. My favourite were the tuna and sweetcorn. Sometimes I was so tired after all of this that I fell asleep in the car on the way home. We tried not to take Mariella, as she wanted a lot of attention and mum and dad needed to concentrate on learning what to do.

Mum and dad seemed pleased about the new injections. We even had a barbeque for all my friends. I didn't even know what mum was up to. She just kept inviting girls around. We had a good time and I was feeling like this might work out a bit better. I was pleased about my new hospital and didn't feel so frightened any more.

CHAPTER TWENTY-FOUR

Holiday in Spain

We went to Alicante for ten days at the end of the school holiday. It was all a bit weird because this was when the airlines had said no to any liquids going in the hand luggage. We had a letter from my Doctor to say that I needed the injections, syringes and creams in the hand luggage

No one even asked mum if she had anything sharp .Our bags went through the x-ray. No one noticed the needles and injections in our hand luggage. They were more worried about having something hidden in my wheelchair. The week before there had been a suspected plot to blow up a plane. More strict guidelines had been brought in.

We went up on a lift whilst I sat in my wheelchair, I could not manage the steps on the plane.

The holiday house was smart; our friends had just left to go home and had left things nice things for us to eat. There was a swimming pool. We spent most of our time in it. We met lots of friends. I found it hard to make friends now as they sometimes don't know about my rotten illness and I can't always join in as I used to. Mum had a quiet word with their mum to explain that I wasn't able to run around the pool etc etc etc etc. Another girl called Rachel arrived. She was good fun. She had a strange accent as she was from Liverpool.

We were having such a good time until it all went wrong. Dad had decided that it would be nice to go to the Irish complex for a change. It was quite a walk and the pavements were well dodgy. Mum was pushing my chair and didn't see the kerb had changed to a downward slope, so she slipped. Dad kept telling her to get up but she looked well bad and was very white. Dad asked me if I could manage to get back to the house, we hadn't come far so I nodded and he helped mum in the wheelchair. She just squeezed in and we went back to the house. Another couple took mum and dad to hospital.

They were gone all day and we stayed with some friends. We had German food .It was not too bad but we were glad to see mum and dad back. Mum came back with a plaster on her arm; she had broken her wrist. We still had a nice holiday and mum did go in the water with the plaster sticking out so it didn't get wet!

CHAPTER TWENTY-FIVE

Year five and my support worker

Mum and dad had told me ages ago that I would be having some help at school. I so didn't want any and I was scared the others would take the mickey out of me and I was not looking forward to it. Mum hadn't said any more about it so I had put it to the back of my mind.

Dad injected my methotrexate now. The nurses showed Mum and Dad how to do it. Mum couldn't do it with her broken wrist so the job has landed on dad.

When the nurse brought the injections round, she asked me if I was looking forward to having some help at school. I was so angry I kicked out at mum and ran upstairs. Was this never ever going to end!

I told mum I wasn't going to speak to my helper at all. I was so upset that I couldn't be normal like the other children. I didn't really speak to her at all at first and she just sat at the back of the class continually calling over 'are you okay Bethany'. I found it really difficult.

When the others were doing stuff that I couldn't do, I spent a lot of time with her – I began to like her, she was very funny. She played for me in games like rounders. She normally ended up on her bum, and this was very funny. I don't think she could be in the Olympics! She does my exercises with me at school and helps with lots of things all the fiddly things that are hard because my fingers are stiff.

We had spent ages in design technology making my doll and I had lots of help to sew it. I was proud of it. The day I bought it home to show mum and dad, Mariella got it and pulled all of the hair out of it. I was very angry so was mum and she had a right go at Mariella. She always wants to ruin my things. Mum says she is jealous but I can't think of any reason why anyone would want to be jealous of me.

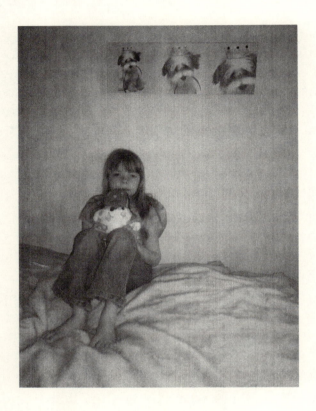

CHAPTER TWENTY-SIX

Winter, colds, aches, and pains

I seemed to have a cold every day through the winter. I always felt tired. When I got a cold about a day later, my joints started to ache then get hot and swell up.

We went shopping, just a quick shop with Mum, Dad and Mariella. I didn't feel good on my feet. Mum had to finish the shop and pay. She found Mariella and I a chair to sit on and I felt a bit better. Mum said that I was as white as a ghost was. I am getting more colds as all the medicine I have are weakening my immune system.

Mum made me have six bits of fruit and veg every day and we had three fruit bowls. I had the orange cod liver oil too. I got lots of mouth ulcers then, but when I had my folic acid, they went away. Mum kept trying to get me to eat more broccoli, which I used to love but my taste buds have changed. Mum couldn't keep up with my varying tastes. One thing I hate having is my tummy medicine. It looks gooey and tastes disgusting but it does stop my stomach aching.

CHAPTER TWENTY-SEVEN

Christmas and Euro Disney

We had a lovely Christmas and Nanny and Granddad came over. I tried out my new knitting machine. We had lots of games and good fun.

On Boxing Day we went to our Nanna's and my auntie, uncle and cousin Amy was there. Mariella was not well that day, mum, and dad had to take her home early. It was nice not having Mariella around moaning for a while.

We all went to Euro Disney with the Brownie group in the middle of January. It was a long way on the coach and we had the back seat so I could stretch out.

I did get very stiff but the driver had to stop for breaks every two hours so I had a stretch out. Two of the girls from school were on the trip and we had a giggle on the way.

When we finally got to Euro Disney, we were tired but excited. We had trouble getting into our room as we were not reading the number on the key properly and we were trying to get into the wrong one. It was funny but I think mum and dad had had enough now. We also left one of our bags on the coach but luckily; Brown Owl had taken it to her room.

The rides were not open as it was late when we finally got out, so we went to Annette's Diner for tea. We had our tea and mum and dad had a glass of wine. This turned out to be very good news for Mariella and me as we went in the Disney shop and mum said 'GO FOR IT' so we went for it. We loaded up our basket and it came to hundreds of euros but lucky for us our nanny and grandad had given us lots of money to spend and we spent it all in about 20 minutes.

When we went into the village the next day it was fantastic even mum was overwhelmed. We all liked the Fantasy World best. Mum made sure we didn't miss the Winter Wonderland show. It was great and was so all so excited.

We got lots of autographs from the characters and everyone working there had to let us on the rides so I didn't have to queue up. Our favourite rides were the Peter Pan and Small World. My favourite character was Minnie Mouse.

I really enjoyed spending time with Mariella, she was a lot of fun on this trip, maybe it's because I was feeling happier that we got on better. We slept in the same bed, there was a big pillow separating us so she didn't accidentally kick me.

Here is a photo of us

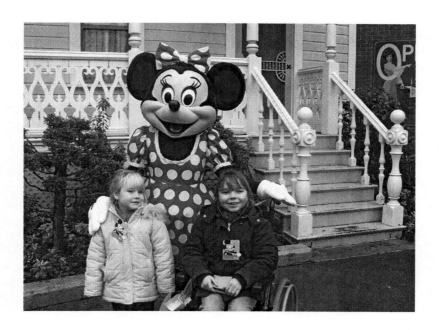

CHAPTER TWENTY-EIGHT

Spring and coming off the steroids

I was still taking the steroids they made my feel better and when I felt sad or tired in the mornings, they would give me some energy and help with my stiffness

I managed to stop taking them a week before we went to Spain. This time it was a bit more organized at the airport and Mum handed over the bag with my syringes and injections in. They didn't open them just put it through the x-ray machine.

We stayed in a bungalow at Rivera-del-sol; it was lovely. There was a pool and a playground and we had a sea-view. There was a bit of a scare about the gas heating though. We had been told not to put the gas on at night. This made Mum and Dad uncomfortable as last year a family had died of carbon monoxide poisoning whilst on holiday. Dad said the bit that took the fumes out was not good enough; it was like our tumble drier hose

We met another family from England. They owned their apartment and they kindly lent us a carbon-monoxide detector. Dad tested the gas, and it was fine, so we just had it on for showers and washing up.

We had another scare on my birthday. It was Dad, he was in the pool and he got into trouble with cramp. Luckily, Mum heard him shout, Mariella and I didn't even hear him. Mum ran and jumped in and pulled him up from the bottom. She couldn't get him out, as he was too heavy. There were only a couple of people around as we were the only ones by the pool, a man came and got him out. He was coughing and spluttering and was much shaken up. It frightened me too, Mariella and me were screaming when they were getting Dad out.

It was my tenth birthday while we were on holiday. I actually got a mobile phone as last. Mum and Dad had promised that we were going to Tivoli World for my birthday treat. It was a theme park about twenty minutes away. I was unsure if we would still go now that Dad had had such a shock.

We did go and had a good time, it was very big and I was tired so I wanted to go in my wheelchair, I thought it would be like Euro-Disney, but it wasn't. It was very difficult to get around and on the rides in my chair.

CHAPTER TWENTY-NINE

My purple evening

We had a purple evening for me at Brownies. Everything was purple, even prizes and gifts. All the money raised was for me, to go towards the hydrotherapy tub.

It was amazing, I went on the cake stall with my friends, and even the cakes had been coloured purple.

I couldn't believe it was for me. My Nanny, Nana, Auntie, Cousin, and some of Mum's friends came along. I don't normally like all this attention and I did get a bit funny when Brown Owl tried to take a photo of everyone, with me at the front. I got a bit overwhelmed and was very tired. Mum made me say thank you to everyone but I didn't want anyone to see me saying thank you. I waited until most people had left.

The next week we were given the cheque. I handed out thank -you notes and sweets to all the Brownies. It wasn't as bad as I had thought having the spotlight on me. Everyone is very kind, especially the Owl's.

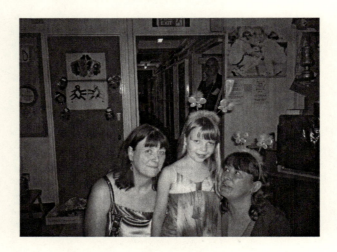

I am feeling a little brighter now. We are not sure why. I have had the methotrexate reduced. I have stopped taking my horrid tummy medicine again and I feel a bit happier. I am getting on better with my little sister, she is kind and caring and sometimes we play together now. She can be very funny. I still get very tired and when I try to do loads of stuff, I normally end up in tears with the tiredness. I get very cold or very hot too. Sometimes I go to bed in two pairs of socks and it's the middle of summer.

I let a little boy who has got Juvenile Arthritis watch me have my injection. He is very frightened having his. I wanted to help him. Mum gave him a sticker to give to me when it had been done. I felt proud of myself for that.

The splints have made my legs straight and I don't have to wear them now that is a relief.

I am going into year six after the summer holiday. What do I hope for in the future? Well to get better would be the first wish and never to have Arthritis again. However, if I do, I suppose my dream would be to do as much as I possibly can and to be happy.

CHAPTER THIRTY

My tips to make things easier

Mum thought it would be a nice thing for me to think of things that would make someone like me feel a bit better so I have come up with some tips:

1. If you hate your splints, try and jazz them up a bit by drawing on them, putting stickers on them or even asking your friends to autograph them.

2. Try to always wear shoes and trainers with Velcro so you don't have to even try to do laces or buckles up.

3. Listen to your favourite music when doing your physiotherapy; it might take your mind off the pain.

4. When things are bad, try to think of things that make you happy and things that you are good at and can still do. Write down or ask someone else to write down all the things you are good at doing.

5. If you feel stiff when sitting down make sure you can stretch your legs.

6. Join a group like the Brownies or Cubs. I love my Brownies and don't want to leave.

7. Try to go swimming or Hydrotherapy sessions if you have a pool nearby, remember that a warm pool makes your joints to relax.

8. The last tip is the most important. You are a star and even if sometimes it all gets too much for you, don't give up on your dreams. Mum says that all this will make me a strong person who can cope with everything. I hope so.

Julie's Journey:

CHAPTER ONE

The nightmare began:

I think we had been let off lightly when Bethany was originally diagnosed with, well what was then called Juvenile Arthritis.

She had hurt her knee when she was two years old. A couple of weeks later it was very swollen and she started to limp, bless her. We weren't that worried to start with and took her to see our GP. He could not feel her knee joint, as her knee was so puffy. She was a little chubby as well so that didn't make it any easier. He decided to refer her to the Orthopaedics' at the local hospital.

When we got there, the Doctor took some x-rays but could not see any bone damage and they did not really know what to do. It started to get a bit more worrying .We were asked to come back for a follow up appointment to see if she had got any better.

Bethany didn't improve. It took six months for her to be referred to a Paediatrician who diagnosed what was then called Chronic Juvenile Arthritis.

We were very surprised as we like most people, didn't even know that children could get Arthritis. She had to have photographs done of her knees and her fingers.

The whole experience seemed bizarre, no one knew what was the matter with her for so long then bang we have a diagnosis. I realise now that other conditions have to be eliminated firstly.

There was a physiotherapist at the appointment. Her name was Ann, and we were going to see her the following week. Mum was with us and Mark my husband at that time wasn't in a job that would allow time off work.

A lady who kept trying to make a conversation with my mum before we went to see the Doctor ran after us as we were going down the stairs. She handed me a brochure. Do you know I could not believe what I was seeing? It was a photograph of a poor physically and mentally disabled child in a wheelchair. I really didn't know what to think at that point.

When we got home, I rang the hospital to try to find out whom the lady was. It was all so overwhelming. I was told that she was a social worker. It was so strange as no one at the appointment had once mentioned that she might want to see us with some information after the appointment.

A long time later, I realised that if that initial meeting had been more professional, she may have been a godsend to as she was from the Lady Hoare Trust. I think if they had contacted us later and said that they could help, it may have been different. However at this point I didn't want any help. Actually, I didn't believe any of it at that point, it all seemed so surreal.

When we went to see Ann at the Children's centre she gave me many exercises to do for Bethany and she checked all her joints.

We were invited to attend the Hydrotherapy sessions. We went a couple of times and I went in the pool with Bethany at this time. Bethany was the only child with Arthritis and the other children were Down's syndrome children.

I found the while experience humbling and at times it felt that I had stepped into someone else's life. I think when you have worried all through your pregnancy hoping and praying that your baby will be healthy, it doesn't dawn on you that they may not stay healthy. I am a lot older and a lot wiser now

Bethany was having terrible side effects to the drugs and was not able to eat she just lay on the sofa lethargically. I had had enough now and told the Paediatrician that she is gripping her stomach in pain. He prescribed her Zantac; I thought the whole thing was out of hand now. She was only three and on drugs that grown ups had

I racked my brains, for ideas to help her and was lucky enough that a friend whose husband was a journalist sent me a video of an item he done on Juvenile Arthritis. Something struck a chord with me. The parents had used homeopathy to help their children. I didn't waste any time and I looked in the yellow pages under the approved homeopath in our area. Luck or fate would have it there was one only a mile away.

We made an appointment and I was amazed at the consultation. Carol asked questions even about the pregnancy and birth and what sort of food Bethany liked and disliked. She made some remedies for her and off we went. Within 24 hours the remedies had worked, I took her off the conventional medicine and was delighted with the results.

However, Bethany's physiotherapist was concerned about Bethany being withdrawn from the drugs without consent from the Doctor. She also told me that Bethany might end up in a wheelchair

I was truly devastated. I thought that they would be pleased that I had found a remedy that was working and that caused no side effects what so ever. What was so nice about the homeopathy was that Bethany was being treated as a whole person and not just a sore knee.

When I got home, I phoned and spoke to the Paediatrician's secretary and told her of my actions. She said she would pass the message onto the Doctor.

I didn't hear anything and knowing what I know now about Bethany's disease, I understand why Ann was so concerned. It seemed, as I was not respecting their judgment. I had little idea of how truly devastating Juvenile Arthritis can be at that time. I had no idea that five years later I was about to find out that the Homeopathy then stood no chance alone.

We continued with the physiotherapy but Bethany came down with a cold after the hydrotherapy and I didn't want to take her back. This was so silly as I was finding it so hard to face up to things and I would say that at this point I was in denial. The puffiness in her knee had reduced and the doctors were pleased.

It was such a shame that I wouldn't let Ann be a support to us as I have spoken to others and she was a complete Godsend to them. I think we had got off on the wrong; she had frightened the life out of me.

The thing is with me, and I do question things if I am not sure. I do find this very uncomfortable as I was brought up in a time where we didn't question anyone let alone a Doctor. Doctors were like God.

However, times have changed and thank goodness, we are now able to have access to information, which in fact gives us a little power over our destinies.

When we went back for the next check up, there were several other doctors in the room. One Doctor in particular was very interested in the Homeopathy remedies that Bethany was taking. What a revelation a Doctor having an interest in Homeopathy however he was much younger and open to new ideas. I explained that Bethany was being treated as a whole person and another child may need different remedies. However, I was pleased that he was interested and was even puzzled by Bethany's progress.

CHAPTER TWO

Life went on

Bethany went to playgroup and was a happy child. She was easy to look after and a joy to be with. She started Nursery and the teacher was aware that she was still attending the hospital for check ups.

When Bethany was four she had an accident at school and this resulted in her left ring and middle fingers being displaced. She had to have surgery and we had a long, long wait for six months to see if the fingertip would take. It was a truly horrible time. My Mum came straight to the hospital to support me. It was such a shock for us to see her fingers in such a state. Luckily, a member of staff had put an ice pack on for her and that had helped.

I stayed in hospital that night with her. We played Monopoly. She has asked for Monopoly ever since. I have only been able to buy it for her this year as it reminded me so much of this awful time.

Bethany began to suffer with anxiety when she went back to school. The bandages had been removed and the fingers didn't look very nice. A couple of the children said how horrible it looked and Bethany started to go to the toilet a lot. This seemed very strange, as this was where the accident happened. However, we were told that this was normal behaviour. The Head teacher spoke to the class about Bethany when she wasn't around and the teasing stopped.

Bethany seemed to do well. We were only going to the hospital once a year to have Bethany's joints checked.

She was discharged from the hospital when she was six. We were told that she was one of the lucky ones, one of the

80% of children that had completely recovered from the Chronic Juvenile Arthritis. Even though she had shown no signs of the disease for some time, we were still delighted and really believed that was the end of it.

CHAPTER THREE

Please don't let this be happening

I was at work at the school nursery. I really loved the job and I felt very lucky to have it. Bethany was at the same school in year three and Mariella at another school nursery whilst I worked.

Whilst I was washing up the children's beakers one day, I happened to glance out of the window. I felt a surge of panic run through my body. Bethany was limping and it was obvious. I looked away hoping that I was seeing things when I looked again she was stood still. It was as if she knew I was watching her.

I found it very hard to concentrate for the rest of the morning. I had mentioned it to one of the girls I work with. I wished the rest of the day away and was very frightened when Bethany came out of school.

I asked her if her left leg was sore, hoping and praying that she may have just hurt herself and that it wasn't going to be anything worse than that. However, her knee was hot and swollen and I reluctantly looked at the rest of her joints. When I looked at her hands, the panic washed over me. I could feel the rush of adrenalin run through my body.. Her fingers were so stiff and she could not bend them.

By the time we got Bethany to see her GP, I had again convinced myself that it was all going to be okay. We had got through the first problem with her knee when she was younger so I did not dream that things were going to turn out so badly for her. The GP was concerned and thought she ought to be referred to the hospital.

Waiting for that appointment was pure agony. Time seem to stand still. I felt so helpless, Bethany had only just told me about the fall she had had in the playground a couple of weeks previously. This really set of the warning bells.

She was prescribed an anti-inflammatory, the same one that caused her such side effects a few years previously. We were told that we would be contacted by the hospital with her appointment date.

CHAPTER FOUR

The Hospital Appointment

It was quite a shock when we got to the hospital appointment. It was the same doctor as Bethany had seen before. However, the other physiotherapist had retired and we met Suzanne, who had replaced her. She was a lot younger and seemed very nice.

Bethany was in a bad way, emotionally and was very anxious when being examined. The Doctor found problems with her thumbs and fingers, they were swollen and she had lost range of movement.

Her knees showed quad wasting, which is wasting of the thigh muscles due to inactivity. Bethany was not using the leg due to the pain. She had loss of range of movement in the right knee. There was also synovial swelling and puffiness of the left knee. Her left ankle was also painful.

We were told that Bethany had extended from an oligo-articular type of juvenile arthritis to a polyarticular phase, which means she has now active disease in more joints. The Doctor advised that she would need to have the anti-inflammatory three times a day and if she didn't respond, she would be a candidate for the disease modifying drug methotrexate. We had to go back in a month for a further review.

Meanwhile, she had photos taken of her affected joints and blood tests, which could give an idea of how much inflammation was in her system.

Bethany really struggled having the photos taken; it was very hard to watch this procedure. She was very down and I was concerned how she was going to cope. Bethany has always been a very bubbly vibrant child, in fact a joy to be around. I really hoped that she was able to deal with all of this.

Mark and I were shocked at the diagnosis. I went straight onto the Internet where I probably spent a large proportion of the next few months.

I was truly obsessed with finding out as much as I could especially about the drug the Paediatrician had mentioned – Methotrexate. I was actually horrified when I found out that Methotrexate was a chemotherapeutic drug used to treat children with Leukaemia.

I felt confused and it took a lot of research for me to understand that it should kill of some off the extra cells that Bethany has in her blood. This should help with the swelling and pain. However, I was very, very concerned reading the possible side affects of the drug. Mood changes, sickness, hair loss, skin rashes.

I felt it was impossible for us to agree to such a powerful drug knowing that it could cause so many future problems.

I made an appointment with my GP for further advice. I was very shocked when I went to see the GP I realised now that he was trying to get through to me how important it was for Bethany to have the Methotrexate. We really had no choice but to agree to it if it was necessary. I knew that she was getting no better at all and that her health was deteriorating before our eyes. I was told that we had to consider her quality of life now and not panic about whether her fertility would be affected in later years

I think that the GP was finding it hard to understand why I was so very against the drug. He told me that if Bethany's condition were left untreated, she would not be able to sustain a pregnancy anyway. I sobbed and sobbed all the way through this very painful revelation. Our daughter was very desperately in need of such a toxic and powerful drug and that I had no choice but to agree to her having them.

That was the worst feeling I had ever felt. I felt that I was letting her down condemning her to a childless future. I knew I had yearned for children so I found it so difficult to imagine life without having children. This is one of the worst parts of her illness. I didn't want her to know about this, I wanted as always to protect her. If I didn't mention it though, it would not really show how difficult it was to make this decision about the drug.

I spoke to my sister on the phone about Bethany. Unfortunately, she was 130 miles away but she had found out about the drug Methotrexate from working in a pharmacy. She knew that I was finding it difficult to agree to Bethany having it and she was anxious that I didn't refuse the drug and frightened the life out of me by saying that she needed to go on it before the disease affected her spine. This was not the first time I had heard of this and I plucked up the courage to ring the boy's mother about their experience on Methotrexate.

She was very understanding, however, she had not had any reservations about the drug. She was more concerned about the effects of the steroids that her son had previously taken at the time. Bethany was not taking any steroids. I was a little surprised that she was not so concerned about the possible side effects. She did confess that he was sick when taking the drug by mouth and when I asked if he had lost any hair, she told me that she had found some on his pillow.

I wonder if it is less frightening for a boy's mother regarding the fertility issue or whether some people have the ability to block out the future and just concentrate on today. I was really struggling with this. I still didn't feel reassured even after speaking to another Mother going through the same issues.

CHAPTER FIVE

The responsibility was overwhelming

Our lives became one of fear. Fear of Bethany being hurt, fear of the drugs, of the future, of everything. It is natural that mothers want to protect their children from pain, however I was not able to.

This really affected my confidence in all areas of my life. I was constantly on edge and unable to relax at all. I really didn't know what to do. We had lost all control over our lives completely. I needed to talk, to ask questions to find out about the future but at the same time, I was terrified to.

Bethany needed a care plan at school so that is when we were introduced to the Community Nursing team.

The first nurse I met tried to reassure me a little and told me that they go to see a little boy with Bethany's condition who lived about ten miles away. He was on the Methotrexate and it was going very well for him. The nurses went in once a week to inject him in the thigh and the medication had really helped. He was described as being a lively little boy doing well.

Karen the nurse could see how worried we were that Bethany was going to be prescribed the Methotrexate so she asked me if I would like to speak to his mum as she may be able to put my mind at rest.

The following day Karen rang and said that the boy's mum was happy to speak to me and gave me her phone number. I put the number in the draw and kept looking at it, I knew I would feel better once I had rung.

I was unable to ring for around three weeks as I was still trying desperately to come to terms with all this. It had happened all happened so quickly over just a week short weeks.

Bethany had gone from a normal mobile girl to a child needing help with everything. She was getting very low in herself and we didn't know what was going to happen ourselves. It was very hard to reassure her. She was so frightened I could hear her sobbing in her bedroom in the mornings.

The mornings were so difficult for her. She was having terrible problems as her leg was seizing up in the night.

At the next appointment with Bethany's physiotherapist, we were told that as Bethany's legs were not straight she would benefit from wearing splints at night. They would also help to prevent her legs seizing up and keep her legs in a resting position whilst she slept. I could remember when she had a splint when she was three.

She was very distressed when having them made before when she was two, and it had to be abandoned. Mum went with her the next day and they managed to make one for her. I found the process very upsetting having to watch helplessly while your child was screaming out. I asked Mark to take her to have the splints made this time, as I knew it was going to be difficult.

The man in the plaster room had not made splints before and Mark said it was awful. Bethany cried out like a Banshee wailing and wailing. The plaster was cold to start with and then it was heated up which was also uncomfortable.

When they brought the splints home I tried to act normal and even made a joke about them. However, I dreaded the night and knew it would be difficult to encourage Bethany to wear them.

CHAPTER SIX

The Swimming Gala

This chapter nearly was forgotten, however it was such a bitter, sweet moment that I needed to add it. Bethany bless her, came home from school and she told me she had entered a swimming gala to be held the following Monday. My mouth must have dropped open and without wanting to hurt her feelings, I said 'what will you be doing exactly'. She said she had entered the relay and the 25-metre race.

I didn't know how to handle this without upsetting her world even more, so I didn't say anything.

I wrote to the school and said that I would come and watch and get her changed. Mark came with us and all the other children were competent swimmers.

Even though Bethany had swum 50 metres doggy paddle style, she had given up lessons as she didn't have the strength and could only just manage a couple of metres.

She was entered in the 10-metre race and she tried her best. She really struggled but she got there. I clapped until my hands were sore. I called her over to ask if she is still going to be in the relay but she had pulled out as another girl had offered to take her place.

It ended on a more positive note as there was a race 25 metres riding a horse (noodle) and this was something Bethany could do as she does this every week in Hydrotherapy.

She done well and almost came in with another couple of children. Well my heart could have burst, we were so proud of her determination; she is such a brave child.

CHAPTER SEVEN

The Loneliness and Isolation

One of the worst feelings was that I now doubted myself in every area of my life. It must be impossible for people on the outside to realise of the sheer torment we were all going. I even felt like the phone had stopped ringing.

The people who I believed would be a shoulder to cry on did not come forward. This not only confused me but also made me withdraw from them.

Bethany was having real trouble walking. We were expecting a wheel-chair buggy to arrive the next day so I was feeling very sad for her.

I had to pop out to the shops and I bumped into someone. They said that I looked miserable. This hurt me so much as this person knew how ill Bethany was. I explained that Bethany's health had deteriorated, but inside I was so angry that I had to justify that I was sad. I was not given an apology. I came home in floods of tears.

This incident was definitely one of many that led to me feeling so alone. My friend came round later and we went out for a meal and a bottle of wine thank God for friends like that.

I was feeling very low in fact; it was more than feeling very low, I was feeling desperate. Mark and I were going through a grieving process for Bethany, you may know what I mean if you are reading this book and your child is unwell.

We cried and cried and grieved for her future as it wasn't looking like a future of choices anymore but one of restriction and uncertainty. I know that parents who have children that are different at birth also go through this process. It is a very lonely feeling and the only other person I felt that was feeling it too was Mark.

CHAPTER EIGHT

Piano Lessons

It was very hard to think of things that would make Bethany feel any better about herself.

She was blaming herself for her illness and said that she was making everyone so unhappy. I knew that my niece was taking piano lessons and found out the number of the tutor from my sister-in-law.

We were very pleased when she said that Bethany could start after the school holidays. Bethany seemed to cheer up when we told her the news.

She was finding it so hard to do anything she loved. Bethany had always been so creative and now she was unable to even hold a pair of scissors.

If I could explain the pain this gave me, it was like having my heart ripped to shreds. I would have swapped places with her a million times over. I was praying for her all the time now that things would start to turn around for her.

My mum seemed to be holding on to the fact that she had recovered before so she may again. However, in her heart, I think she knew that this time was so very, very different.

Our homeopath was still sending remedies however the vile disease was not going to shift this time.

One of Bethany's friend's dad has described her illness as being evil and that is just what it was- pure and utter evil.

I do not know how I was expected to carry on as before. Nothing in my life was as it was before; my whole being was now wrapped up with looking after Bethany.

Mark had adapted the taps around the house and put a bath rail in. She still needed help but this did give her a little more independence. Bethany was using adult disabled cutlery, which she hated. She has designed some cutlery suitable for children and beakers that would be easier to hold for children with difficulties with grip. I hope one day that we can do something with those designs, that we can find someone to help her, so that children like Bethany can hang onto some dignity. She is such a creative child.

CHAPTER NINE

Methotrexate

Bethany started middle school. They were armed with care plans and Ibroprofen to give her at lunchtime. We had had a meeting with the school and Karen; one of the Community nurses came. Karen in fact is still in our lives and to me is one of those special people who I am sure is an angel in disguise

It was agreed that Bethany would not have to go out at playtimes. She could stay in with a friend and that she at the time would not have to do PE or games either.

Two days after Bethany started her new school, we had the follow up appointment with the Paediatrician.

We told him about the past few weeks and how Bethany was finding it difficult to open her mouth and get around. When he examined her, he found arthritis in her jaw; she had painful stiff fingers, knees, and also right hip and elbow.

He advised that she would need to have some more aggressive medication to control her inflammatory arthritis-Methotrexate. This was the news that we knew was inevitable. We were told that she would be on this drug for one or two years. We were told that Bethany would need monthly blood tests, that Methotrexate was an immunosuppressant, and that Bethany should not have live vaccines while she was on it. Bethany was thankfully fully immunized and had had chicken pox.

We were told that should her blood tests show significant neutopenia, low platelets or abnormalities of liver function, and then I would be informed immediately to stop the Methotrexate. This was extremely unusual in children where tolerance is greatest and toxicity much rare than in adults. We were also told that they have gratifying results from the use of Methotrexate in paediatric arthritis with very satisfactory long-term outcomes.

Bethany was also prescribed a higher dose of Ibuprofen. In addition, she was prescribed Losec/Omeprazole as additional gastric protection and we were told that he would see her again in a month's time.

We were given the prescription for the Methotrexate and that was that. However, it was not as straight forward as that. Even obtaining the Methotrexate was a complete nightmare.

We went to our local pharmacy and they did not stock it and in fact had never heard of it being prescribed to a young child. This only added to the anguish of having to give it to her. Mark took the prescription back to the hospital pharmacy; he was finally given the drugs.

Bethany really tried to take the tablets however bearing in mind that she now had active arthritis in her jaw; she found it impossible to swallow. This was now becoming a huge issue for us and Bethany was very distressed.

I told the community Nursing Team that Bethany was unable to swallow the tablets. A nurse arranged to come round and help us. The nurse seemed a little anxious in handling the Methotrexate and explained to us that we must not touch it. It is just medicine for Bethany only and if anyone touched it could seep through our skin and affect our blood cells. This was almost unbelievable. Bethany was noticing the fact that the nurse had gloves on and that she would not touch the medicine. I really do not blame her that she was not keen to take it either. She started gagging and it all became so very uncomfortable. I suggested that she may be better having the injection instead and was amazed to be told that I was looking for an easy way out. This was quite difficult to absorb.

I would say at that point in our lives things were as far removed from easy as could possibly be.

The whole Methotrexate issue was now becoming larger than life itself. However, the pediatrician agreed to prescribe the injections. Every Thursday one of the three nurses would come round and inject her in the thigh. We put on the magic cream to numb the area around 45 minutes before they were due to arrive.

The side effects of the Methotrexate really came into force around three weeks later.

Bethany's moods were very bizarre and she didn't seem to be able to control the very low periods. The night sweats started and Mark and I took it in turns to wipe her down with a cold flannel. She was burning hot, bearing in mind that she was wearing two splints from her knee to her ankles as well. Mark installed a ceiling fan and we had this on full power for her. It was October now so it was not the height of summer.

Then the night terrors started. I would only explain this as watching a child hallucinating. It was unbearable to watch. It always seemed to be about the same thing. She would scream that she was growing another tooth but she described the tooth as more of a tusk. It was such a relief that she did not ever remember these episodes the next day.

Mark and I were just never getting a break from it now. Being awake intermittently in the night was now becoming a real problem.

I kept questioning what we were doing giving her this drug and all the time waiting for the 'quality of life' to arrive. I was constantly on the Internet looking at websites about Juvenile Arthritis and its treatments- especially the Methotrexate. However, nothing I read set my mind at rest in fact it was just the opposite. I had read that it was used for terminations. I couldn't get my head around how it worked and knew that it was toxic so in my mind that made it the enemy to start with. How could it know which cells to kill each week, well the reality was it could not and Bethany's symptoms now started to vary considerably.

CHAPTER TEN

My Meltdown

It is probably obvious to anyone reading this that I was in a bad way. I was so trying to keep on going without changing the rest of my life. However, it was impossible to carry on.

I was going to work and doing a reasonably good job of hiding up the pain and sorrow, I felt. However, one day at work, I was just about to go home and an incident happened. Something and nothing, but I ended up in tears. Once the tears came they didn't stop. It was as if I just couldn't ask anyone to do anything for me, I think that was how I was feeling about home. It was spilling out in every area of my life.

I went and saw my GP and he signed me off work for a month. He explained how all the recent events had now caught up with me and that I needed a break.

I was later told that the others were worried that I was going to collapse in the corner with exhaustion. The events that happened later that day really showed how much of a break I needed.

I had been given a phone number from work, a wellbeing phone line. I was now desperate that I intended to ring and see what was on offer.

CHAPTER ELEVEN

The Hospital Admission

The very same day that I had been signed off work, Bethany became unwell, she had a bad sore throat. I took her to see our GP who at the time was on holiday so we saw one of the locum GP's.

She checked Bethany's throat and took her temperature. She was feverish. The doctor asked if Bethany had had any other blood tests whilst being on Methotrexate and I said that she had not. With that, she was on the phone to the Children's ward at the local hospital saying that she was sending her up straight away. I panicked. I had Mariella to consider and the doctor was extremely concerned about Bethany.

I managed to find a friend at home. He drove us up to the ward and meanwhile contacted Mark at work.

Bethany was given a bed and I was asked many questions about her health that week. They took some blood tests, which she found very distressing and she screamed and screamed. A tourniquet caused the most of the pain. They do not have to use one anymore, thankfully. We had quite a wait before a doctor came. He explained that Bethany had an infection and a fever. He reassured us that the blood tests were not showing any neutropenia, low platelets or abnormalities of the liver, which was a huge relief.

We had to wait until eleven o'clock that night before they would let her go home and do you know what, we were still waiting for the 'quality of life'. Looking at my child's pale thin face and seeing how frightened she was, I again questioned the Methotrexate.

I was relieved that I could take work out of the equation now for four weeks, as things had become so out of control. I did take up the offer of counselling. I was now feeling so vulnerable. I had four sessions. It was very helpful and brought to light how difficult it was for me to ask for help. I found myself crying throughout the sessions but it did me good and helped me regain some strength to continue.

CHAPTER TWELVE

Follow up appointment

Bethany had a follow up appointment the next month. The doctor examined Bethany and said that she had some spindling deformities of the small finger joints. She did not have full grip and the quad wasting needed a lot of work. He also said that the CRP was 31 and that still was an ongoing inflammatory process. She needed to be reviewed again in a month's time.

It was extremely difficult to accept that your child had spindling deformities, you did not feel like smiling or laughing, it was distressing.

We were now finding it so difficult to talk to the Doctor or anyone else about how she really was not coping. If I said for example that she needed help with things like squeezing toothpaste, Bethany would give me a scowl or even actually kick me.

When we left, the appointment things got worse and she acted as if I had betrayed her.

I really did not know which way to turn now and I was starting to feel like I was closing up as well and all I wanted to do was hide away. I was not finding anyone to share this.

Mark was also so stressed. Some friends were managing to ask how things were. That meant a lot to me although I think, as it was almost impossible for them to put themselves in our shoes. It was almost inevitable that they would say something inappropriate without meaning to.

My parents were finding it very difficult and were upset at Bethany's plight. Mum kept hoping for a miracle and was always finding out about complementary therapies for Bethany to try. She brought her a cool chill pillow, which was nice wrapped around her ankles at night.

Mum suffers from Osteoarthritis in her knee. This is wear and tear of the joints, this condition is very different to Bethany's however, but the pain is the same. Mum also has acupuncture, which she finds helpful. I have had a course of acupuncture myself for hay fever and I did find it helpful.

I asked Bethany if she would try reflexology or see a Chinese practioner but she refused. In fact, she was refusing point blank now to talk about much at all. I still think to this day that she needs to have the energy in her body realigned and hope that she will come round to this idea.

I am so grateful for my parent's help through all of this, Mum is tirelessly always looking for new ways to help Bethany.

Bethany's frame of mind was so altered I hardly recognised her. She was now a sad, sullen, snappy and very sad little girl. She was finding it impossible to interact with anyone and was constantly going off in a huff, something she had never done before.

I would say that Bethany was a most agreeable, pleasant child before all this started. Everyone was saddened at how despondent she now was.

If I mentioned how much the drugs and of course, the disease was affecting her, it was shrugged off as her age. This was completely untrue and it made me cross that no one would even discuss the side effects with me.

I began to feel quite indignant that my child was being disregarded. I had to fight now to be heard. However, there were decent people who could see her suffering. It was not easy to spot especially if you only saw a brief window of her day. Bethany had become quite an actress now. She was so determined to hide her pain and distress, she was not able to flush the toilet and Mark and I just went in after her without saying anything. We did not make any fuss over the things she could not do.

She sometimes looked pleadingly at me for me to help her with one task or another, which broke my heart.

CHAPTER THIRTEEN

Methotrexate increasing

When we went back the following month, Bethany was examined again and we were advised that objectively there was little change. The ESR (Erythrocyte Sedimentation Rate) was 26. The Doctor thought that she was turning the corner but suggested stepping up the Methotrexate to 12.5mg from 10mg. So in fact, it was to be increased 25%. He asked to see her again in January, which was two months later.

Mark and I were amazed again at the news. The Methotrexate was to be increased; we were dreading the night sweats and terrors becoming worse as well.

Bethany was managing to keep the splints on a little longer but some nights she could only cope with one of them on. She was working hard on the punishing regime of daily physiotherapy and the weekly Hydrotherapy. Bethany looked forward to the hydrotherapy, as it was there that she got a chance to meet other children and I other parents.

The whole experience on a Friday morning was almost humbling. Mark and I found it so draining emotionally to see the disabled children in a group.

The therapy workers were lovely and at last, I found someone to talk with. Sandy took her time to listen whilst she passed the toys into the pool. I think she knew how bad things were for us. She is a respite worker herself and suggested that we needed a break. She was right but Bethany was not able to relate to anyone other than us, so it was impossible for others to meet her needs.

The grandparents did take both girls out and they had been taking turns in taking Bethany to hydrotherapy while I worked. I gave up my Friday morning when I returned to work so that I could take Bethany to Hydrotherapy. She had to come first.

When Bethany and Mariella went out, together, Bethany she was reluctant to use the buggy, so Bethany was carried about. This had a detrimental effect on Mariella as she was really feeling left out now.   Poor Mariella, she was going to school each day and seemed to be doing okay with her work. It took her a long time to make a friend and she was very, very quiet.

We were all focusing on Bethany that we had somehow forgotten how much Mariella was missing out on. It was quite funny, as every time Mariella saw me she said she was hungry regardless of how much she had just eaten. I think it was her little way of getting attention.

CHAPTER FOURTEEN

The Christmas Show

Bethany wanted to join in with the Danz Kidz show being held at the local holiday centre. She tried to join in with a few of the dances, bless her she could not even bend down but she was so determined to have a go.

When the show was over, I was so proud of her that I wanted to go and grab the microphone and announce to everyone what an achievement that had been for her.

She was exhausted when we got home but I know it did her the world of good. She was stuck on the outside of her life just looking in most of the time. This time she was part of something.

That Christmas was a little more relaxed. We managed to have friends over and even had a few laughs. Mum and Dad came over and we all had lunch.

Bethany was not able to sit on the floor so we had to play games on the table. Our dog Honey was a pain anyway if anything was left on the floor she would take it and chew it to pieces.

We tried to make it a nice Christmas and we went to see Mark's mum on Boxing Day with his sister, brother-in-law and Niece. It was nice to go out, we had not been out much at all over the last eighteen months.

Bethany still did not want anyone to see her in her buggy and she was not able to walk. So normal life was put on hold.

It felt like we were prisoners in our own home. I did not think that Bethany was ever going to come to terms with her disability and that made me very sad. I told her of others that were in much worse situations and she did understand, but it gave her no comfort. I suggested that we went to a hospice but she found that too much to cope with.

CHAPTER FIFTEEN

Hospital again

After Christmas, we had another appointment to check on Bethany's progress with the pediatrician.

He was still insisting that her grip was normal. However she was not actually able to use her hands or fingers at all and it must have taken every ounce of her being, to have grasped his fingers with such might. It was a sad sight to us as she was only harming herself by hiding her true plight.

The pediatrician was not seeing the true picture. He suggested that she might need to have the Methotrexate increased again in future, as the ESR was still at 28. As Bethany was having trouble with the Losec, he suggested that we could now reduce the Ibuprofen by 50% for a week and then stop; this would mean that she would no longer need the stomach protection of the Losec mups.

We went ahead and to our horror, Bethany was no longer mobile She was in a lot of pain so we spoke to the Community Nurse who passed on a message that we had resumed the Ibuprofen.

It all seemed to be such an experiment. We had told the school to stop the lunchtime medicine and I had to go down again and sign the forms for it all to be started up again.

At this point, Mark and I were starting to feel very edgy about her treatment. We could have done with some kind of support group, someone to help us. It was that we felt alone in that people were not talking to us about Bethany or how we were coping. Not all people and the ones who were there were truly appreciated. I hope they know that.

We received silence if we mentioned Bethany so we had to pretend it was not happening - it was all so bizarre. The best thing I could have done at that point was to have mixed with others in a similar predicament whom would understand the sorrow we were feeling.

CHAPTER SIXTEEN

The car accident and downward spiral

As our lives had been so wrapped up in Bethany and not much else, I racked my mind to think of something we could do in the Easter holidays.

Mark had booked off a long weekend and I had been in touch with an old school friend who I hadn't seen for a number of years who was still living in Hertfordshire about twenty miles away from where we grew up. We planned to go and see Heather and her daughter Kirsten who was our bridesmaid 11 years previously.

We had also planned to meet up with other relatives. I had found a Travelodge with a heated swimming pool. It would be great for Bethany and in fact for all of us to have a swim and relax. It all sounds nice doesn't it?

We travelled down to Hertfordshire with no problems, despite Bethany getting very stiff in the car. We had breaks on the way and arrived at around one o'clock. It was great to see Heather. We had been firm friends all the way through school from the age of four. The new house was great; it was a struggle for Bethany to get to the top though.

We had lunch then decided to head back to the travel lodge. We were driving around a large roundabout at St. Albans when a car had hit us. The woman got out of the car and started shouting and screaming although it was obviously her fault as she had been changing lanes and did not see us. Mark had to reverse the car back as her bonnet was stuck into the driver's door. She became so abusive that whilst Mark tried to calm her down I ended up ringing 999. I spoke to the police and they gave me advice, as she was not going to produce her insurance details before I rang them. I was in shock now but managed to hold things together. I told her to stop shouting, as one of my children was sick. This seemed to bring her back to reality and she apologised for the accident and said that she hoped my daughter would soon be better. She drove off and somehow Mark managed to get us to the hotel

Bethany had not spoke through this very disturbing incident. I felt so responsible for her, how could this have happened we came away to try to have some normality and to take our minds away from her illness.

We thought that a swim would be good I noticed that Bethany was unable to raise her arm and knew that the accident had caused a problem in her shoulder. Not only did I now feel sick, I actually felt the lowest I had felt in my whole life.

We had dinner although I could not eat and Mark was very low too. We tried to settle the children to sleep early evening so we could talk about the accident. However, we were all awake until two in the morning.

We set off the next morning to meet my sister and brother-in-law at Willow Farm. Bethany had stiffened up a lot and when we got to there she was very tearful and we could see that she was unable to walk.

We offered to get her buggy out so she could relax and enjoy the day. However, she could not cope with this and Mark ended up carrying her on his shoulders all day. She only weighed about two and a half stone at this time so it was not too bad. Mark put a brave face on, as he was experiencing pain in his shoulders too from the accident. My neck seemed very awkward too but I just shrugged it off. When you have a child in so much pain, it feels inappropriate to moan about trivial things yourself.

We had a nice day and decided rather than stay another night in the Travel lodge, we should head home. The children really needed their own beds.

Mark went to the GP when we got home and was told he had whiplash. He had some physiotherapy to help this. I was uncomfortable too but had to concentrate on Bethany. She was not able to talk about the accident and started screaming if it was mentioned. I knew it would be a waste of time taking her to be looked at so I dropped a letter into our GP to inform him of the accident and that I had stepped up the Physiotherapy.

At the next hydrotherapy session, I quietly told Suzane about the accident so she could surreptitiously check her joints in the hydrotherapy pool.

CHAPTER SEVENTEEN

A turn for the worse

Within two weeks, Bethany had started to have major problems not only in her joints. She was almost shuffling along and it was the most frightful sight to see.

She was unable to talk at all now; she had completely retreated into herself. If I tried to talk to her and try to see the best way to care for her, she would kick and scream out and run to her bedroom. This had a detrimental effect on all of us.

Our marriage by now was hanging on a thread and Mariella seemed to be behaving like a baby. Mariella was still wetting the bed although she was four. She was acting very inappropriately. Although we knew in our hearts that seeing her sister suffer, so much was very traumatic for her. We did not know how to help her.

Bethany was refusing to leave her bedroom and was now hiding in her wardrobe rather than face up to the illness. It was truly heartbreaking.

Her weight seemed to plummet and she looked desperately ill. When the nurses and the physiotherapist saw Bethany, they were concerned. The nurse tried to track down the Paediatrician at the hospital to tell him of Bethany's plight, however, he was on holiday.

Bethany was using her piano as a lifeline. She was talking about killing herself and about how useless she was. I started to get angry that my innocent daughter was just being left in such a bad way.

Karen and Bethany's physiotherapist Suzanne and I went to a meeting at Bethany's school. Bethany was not coping and they didn't know what to do.

Bethany's teacher said that he was asking her if she was okay and she was just nodding and smiling but of course, she was far from okay. Suzanne, the physiotherapist said she could do with some physiotherapy within school time especially in the morning when she was so stiff. It was out of the question before school as she was immobile for the first two hours.

Bethany needed some help during lessons. The fact that she was not able to flush the toilet was also becoming an issue. They had not been able to persuade her to use the disabled facilities.

We agreed that the school would apply for some special funding for Bethany.

CHAPTER EIGHTEEN

The smile has dropped

The following Monday I was paying for my shopping in the supermarket when my mobile rang .It was Bethany's school.

Bethany was screaming and crying, they had never seen her like this before, and they wanted me to go to see her. I was getting used to seeing her like this nearly every day.

When I arrived, Bethany was in the medical room in a bad way. She was very obviously distressed and it was a difficult to find out what had happened.

Her teacher had tried to help Bethany by telling the class that if Bethany left the classroom she was going to do some exercises she wasn't going to Mrs Hall's set. The mere mention Mrs. Hall's set had sent Bethany berserk. Mrs. Hall took the children who had special requirements and Bethany had been terrified that her classmates would think that she had become less able to do her work.

I had to calm her down. The only thing that worked was the homeopathic remedy. It took a minute or two and then she was able to understand that her teacher was just trying to reassure her. He was upset to see her in such a state.

This was the first time someone else had seen her being so distressed. Bethany refused to do any exercises at school. She was in such a state that we had to postpone the exercises until we could talk her round.

How she was ever going to cope with a support worker I really do not know. Again, she was making me feel that again I was betraying her.

CHAPTER NINETEEN

It is all out of control –
The piano starts to talk

Things were now out of control, out of our control and certainly out of Bethany's control – it was very unnerving.

When I feel out of control, I revert to an old pattern of strict dieting a habit, which started when I was a teenager. I was finding it hard to keep a grip and was yet again denying myself food as a way of control. It was very difficult for me having to continually fight Bethany's corner.

Playing the piano seemed to calm Bethany down. When she was frustrated, she banged the keys down in such a dark loud way. One day when she was playing, I asked her to play me how she felt. It was quite moving. She was actually talking to me through her piano. I had to act fast and asked her to play the notes to describe her pain on a scale of 0-10. She started to respond and I was getting a picture of which of her joints were causing the most pain and how she felt about her illness.

When Bethany and Mariella had gone to bed, I told Mark about the breakthrough and we both sobbed and sobbed. Our child, she was born so perfect and now is such pain. We felt so HELPLESS.

CHAPTER TWENTY

My friend – a friend indeed

I was sitting in the staff room at coffee break and I happened to switch on my mobile. We are not allowed to have them on in the Nursery. I was about to text a friend when I noticed that I had a text from my friend Vicki who was working at another school. She told me that there was going to be a speaker from the University of East Anglia at the school tonight and the subject was going to be Arthritis.

At that time I had no idea how that text was going to change our lives for the better.

Vicki came and picked me up. The meeting was predominately about Osteo-Arthritis, which is the wear and tear that normally occurs in later life. However, when he briefly spoke about his patients with Rheutomtoid Arthritis how they were benefiting from the new anti-tnf drug. I sat up and became very interested. I gathered all my nerves together and asked if children would benefit from the anti-tnf drugs. He nodded. This was now sounding positive, the first piece of positive news we had heard for a long time.

I told him about Bethany and the fact that the Methotrexate was no longer able to control the activity and even told him that she was not RF factor but ANA factor.

After the meeting, he told me that we needed to see a Rheumatologist at the Norfolk and Norwich hospital to assess Bethany. He even thought that we could pay for a private consultation and then she would be taken on as a patient. This was music to my ears. I told him that we had an appointment with Bethany's pediatrician the following day and he told me to ask for a referral. I knew that I was going to do this whether I felt intimidated or not. I could not allow this to continue, not even for one more day.

CHAPTER TWENTY-ONE

We want a referral please

Bethany's community nurse had arranged to inject Bethany with the Methotrexate at the hospital before her appointment. We had made this arrangement by text. I texted her to say that Bethany was not any better. I also mentioned my plans to ask for a referral to a Rheumotologist.

She was such an angel and she said she would come to the appointment with us.

Just before, we went in. Karen told me that she had told the pediatrician that I was going to ask for a referral. He agreed to send a report to a rheumatologist called Dr Armon asking for a second opinion.

It is quite important to mention that she always saw this pediatrician late in the afternoon, which actually is normally the best time for children with Arthritis as the medication, has kicked in and the joints have loosened up.

CHAPTER TWENTY-TWO

Waiting and waiting in despair

We waited and waited but there was still no news from the hospital. When I asked I was told they had yet to receive the referral. I chased the secretary at the original hospital who agreed to send another fax.

I could not let this rest now and rang our GP who was very encouraging. He said were within our rights to have a second opinion and he would also send a referral and ask for Bethany to be seen privately if necessary as things were so bad for us at home.

Bethany was having panic attacks about seeing another doctor. Unbelievably someone actually questioned whether we should leave her alone as she was obviously so traumatised. How could I not stop trying to find the best care for her? I was not going to let her down and if there was a drug out there that would make any improvements to her life, then she deserved it. Do not forget we were still waiting for her 'quality of life' to improve through the Methotrexate

I discussed the appointment at work as I was now getting worried. My colleagues suggested that I could fund raise for Bethany to pay for the drug if needed. I hoped it would not come to that as by now I was running on empty. I had done some research and had found that it would cost around £12,000.00 a year for the anti-tnf drug. Entanacept (trade name embrel) is a type of drug known as an anti-tnf (anti-Tumor Necrosis Factor). In people and children with arthritis, a protein called TNF is present in the blood and joints in excessive amounts where it increases inflammation

My GP was sure that if Bethany qualified for it, she would not be refused on the grounds of cost. With that information, we were ready.

CHAPTER TWENTY-THREE

Please give my child back her childhood

We had an appointment the Consultant Pediatric Rheumatologist on Tuesday 13 June 2006; she was going to see Bethany on the Children's Ward. We were delighted .At last and I felt that Bethany was going to see a doctor who had experience with children who have not responded to the other drugs.

Bethany almost hobbled along when we got there and we were introduced to Dr Kate Armon and to Kit, a specialist nurse in Rheumatology. I did not realize that there were such nurses. We also met the physiotherapist.

Dr Armon discussed the current treatment and the reason for the referral. I went through everything that had happened and how Bethany had coped with the drugs and all the difficulties she was having. I found it all very emotionally draining. I felt like Bethany's future was in this doctor's hands and if she could not see how ill she was-well I could not even go there. I could feel myself welling up, and I was sobbing and sobbing.

I told the doctor that Bethany had lost a year of her childhood .I almost begged her to help.. I asked her to consider her for the new anti-tnf drug. Dr Armon just nodded and said that she would help her. They were the best words I had heard in my whole life. I pulled myself together and Bethany was then examined.

This examination was very different to all the other examinations. We knew that she could see the pain she was suffering. Bethany had been weighed and measured and she was the weight of a baby. She weighed just over two and a half stone. She was painfully thin and her legs were like matchsticks.

I was very surprised at hear the Doctor say that she would like to admit Bethany for intravenous Methulprednisolene. She would need to stay in for two nights. We agreed but the look on Bethany's face told a different story.

Kit took Bethany to the ward and showed her the beds and equipment but Bethany started crying and kicking out. I told her that I could stay in with her but that did not help. She was so traumatised by this stage and her knees were so swollen I think that she could not take anymore. I asked the doctor if I could give her homeopathic remedy to calm her down and she agreed. Within minutes, Bethany calmed down and Dr Armon agreed that if Bethany could keep down 40mg of Prednisolone a day, she could go home. Bethany grabbed this lifeline and took the medicine.

We were advised that the dose could drop to 20mg then 10mg. (Prednisolone is a form of steroids. They help with the inflammatory process and immune response. Steroids stop the normal production of cortisone from the adrenal glands and MUST be taken regularly. This means that doses should only be changed gradually to allow the gland to recover. Children will be issued with an official card so that in case of accidents, other people can see that they need to continue to take their oral steroids. There can also be a poorer absorption of calcium, which can lead to osteoporosis. So, they encourage the children to eat more calcium rich foods like milk.)

Dr Armon's assessed Bethany. Her height was 121.cm, weight 19.66kg (0.8m2), blood pressure 112/74, and pulse 115. She had a soft systolic murmur. This was news to us. Musculoskeletal examination revealed marked involvement of all DIPJ'S and PIPJ'S, thumbs and CMC joints, wrists, knees and subtler joints. There was significant effusion, warmth and limited mobility. She noted that Bethany was pale and fairly miserable. Her height was plotted on the 2nd centile; her weight to the 0.4th centile.

Although Bethany had been on a good dose of Methotrexate, she was still suffering from very active disease. The blood test showed an ESR of 53, Haemoglobin 11, white blood cells count 10, platelets 497.

We spent the rest of the day at the hospital. Kit stayed with us and pushed Bethany around in a wheelchair. She had to have x-rays to be allowed to go ahead with the anti-tnf drug-Entanacept.

Kit was so supportive and Bethany seemed to relate to her. It was nice to see her talk openly to a medical person. Kit is a guider and as Bethany goes to Brownies, they had something in common, something positive.

Dr Armon discussed Entanacept, one of the anti-tnf drugs and gave us information sheets to read and we had a start date of July 7th. Anti-tnf drugs have to be given by subcutaneous injections (an injection under the skin) twice a week.

This was the best news ever. Bethany was going to have the best drug available and her care now involves a nurse trained in rheumatology. She would be able to answer and guide us through. We had been told that we would need to make a huge commitment as we needed to travel to the hospital twice a week to be trained on injecting the Entanacept which would eventually be delivered to our home

Mark was able to take time off work. In fact, the hours lost where given back to him because he was caring for a sick child. It was great that Mark's employers were so supportive.

CHAPTER TWENTY-FOUR

The Echocardiogram

Just after the first visit to see Dr Armon, I was suddenly struck with a sense of panic about the heart murmur.

I got straight onto the Internet and found out to my horror, that Arthritis can affect the heart. I was completely shocked.

I sent and email to the hospital to clarify. I had a reply straight away and Dr Armon tried to reassure me that finding the murmur was incidental, however as it can be part of the disease, we need to have it checked out. It would be treated with Prednisolene. I felt helpless again, why didn't we know about the murmur before?

Meanwhile, we did not have to wait long for the appointment and it was on a Friday.

Mariella had obviously picked up on the stress. When she woke up and she told Mark that she could not walk. I do not think for a minute that Mark would have taken it so seriously if he were not so anxious about the appointment later that day. I suppose after what we have been through with Bethany, nothing would surprise us anymore. I went to see Mariella. She put on a good performance. The whole episode was sad to watch. I managed to trick her into walking and tried to make her feel a bit better. She is so jealous of the attention Bethany gets. The funny thing is Bethany just does not want any attention. It was a lose, lose situation.

We finally got Mariella to school and set off for the 26-mile journey to the hospital. We only had 10 miles when the phone rang. It was Mariella's school. Had she convinced them she couldn't walk as well. I took the call and blurted out 'was it her legs'. No, she had a weepy eye and they were convinced it was conjunctivitis. I panicked, as we could not turn back. Luckily, my parents-as ever-were able to pick her up.

When we got there, I told Mark I couldn't face it. I was so worried. Mark was brilliant and took her in.

I sat waiting dreading my little baby having further problems. They were not too long, but it felt like I had waited forever. Mark came out with the report and said she had a small murmur, nothing too serious. I felt so very grateful and thanked God and Bethany's guardian angel. Dr Armon met us, took the report, and said it was fine. Again, a feeling of huge relief washed over me.

CHAPTER TWENTY-FIVE

Training on Entanacept (enbrel)

When we had training on the drug, we were given handouts and had the side affects advised to us.

We were told that Bethany should not inhale passive smoke as the cells in her lungs will be altered with the drug and that her liver would not be able to withstand alcohol. This was not a problem for us as neither of us smoked; I had smoked for ten years but had given up 16 years ago.

We were advised that no one knows the affect of Entanacept on an unborn baby so as Methotrexate, sustaining a pregnancy on these drugs would be out of the question.

We had agreed that Bethany could take part in a research study as its vitally important for more information on the side effects of enbrel because it has not been in use for very long.

In addition, Bethany had agreed to be part of a study being done by a medical student and doctor through the t Medical School at the University. They were in particular looking at the blood tests that monitor the arthritis, the swelling and other factors which may affect the blood tests. They were also looking at the ESR and CRP tests to try to establish if one was better than the other was at recording the physical signs of arthritis such as sore swollen joints and limited mobility.

These blood tests were taken every four weeks for children on these drugs and the results are closely monitored. Bethany was hesitant at first thinking that she would have to have another person examine her. I explained that it would be all done through her file at the hospital and

99

she wouldn't know anything about it. I also pointed out to her how important it was for the medical team to know which tests are more reliable.

Kit said that Bethany would benefit from some play therapy sessions, which could start the following week. I could not believe it. Not only were professionals seeing her plight, they were in a position to actively help.

We went to the hospital twice a week and Bethany bonded with both Kit and Judy the play worker. It was lovely to see her chatting a little more. She enjoyed the sessions with Judy although she would not talk about her illness and how it affected her. I think that we had hoped she would come to terms with it a bit more and be able to speak out. It was, and still is difficult to look after a child when they will not tell you how much pain they are in. Mark and I can always spot Bethany's difficulties because she adapts the way she does things if a joint is sore.

Sometimes she finds it easier to skip than walk. What others may see as a sign of joy is actually a sign that she is struggling.

Rather than ask for help, Bethany will trick you into doing something for her. She has become quite a little actress. When a professional faces her, she will put on quite a performance to hide how she really is.

We have now come to terms with the fact that Bethany has the right not to talk about it and we do not press her anymore.

It would have helped her so much to have had a friend with Arthritis, but although I was very hopeful when I joined the Contact a Family) on the website.

We only found one other girl Bethany's age also on the Entanacept but she lived in New Zealand - you could not have anywhere much further away could you? I'm sure the system works well with some people we were just unlucky.

CHAPTER TWENTY-SIX

What about Mariella?

Throughout summer, Bethany was our focus. We were travelling to and from hospital and taking in all the instructions so we could prepare and inject the Enbrel.

We managed to go on holiday but I broke my wrist and that then caused major problems. I couldn't push Bethany's wheelchair to school. We had to rely on friends and family to help us.

As Mariella had achieved her targets in reception, I was not too worried that we had not spent much time with her over the summer and thought that she would do okay going into Year 1.

It was not until I went to see her teacher for parents evening that I was put in the picture. When I saw her work, I was shocked. She had written her letters and words back to front. She was having problems in all areas and her confidence was very low.

The teacher had given her an individual Education plan. I was mortified. The guilt hit me like a ton of bricks – how had this happened?

I felt so responsible. I didn't know when I was going to manage to help her. I really had no spare time. Bethany's care took up hours. I just cried, cried, and really made such a show of myself. When I got home, I told Mark and he too was upset. We now had two children that needed extra time and we were already struggling so much to fit everything in. We knew that Mariella was quite able so it must have been her self-esteem and confidence. Apparently, she had been very quiet in the class.

So we spent hours with her, I spent hours with her reading and going over the work they were covering. If she saw a word she did not recognise, she would sob and sob. I knew that we needed to make her feel better about herself. Somehow, we had to help her with her confidence.

The school was fantastic. The teacher had looked up her reception work and seen the difference. Mariella and a small group of other children went to nurturing sessions. She is slowly being more confident. However, we have a long way to go with her.

It is very hard on a sibling in this situation. Bethany was in so much pain, if Mariella knocked into her, that she screamed. It was so hard on Mariella to be told to be careful around Bethany. When Bethany feels very low, this has a knock-on effect to Mariella and to us all. We certainly felt that we were failing to meet Mariella's needs.

The unpredictable nature of Bethany's illness absorbed so much of our time, energy and emotion.

CHAPTER TWENTY-SEVEN

My acceptance a long time coming

Its now almost two years ago, that Bethany started limping. We have all been on a journey, a very long and exhausting journey and one that we are still continuing.

Bethany is still having the Methotrexate, and Entanacept injected into her thigh. She is having the most problem with the methotrexate as it stings so much. She also has for pain Piroxicam, Lansoprazole to help with the stomach problems, weekly folic acid, which helps with mouth ulcers.

We are weaning her off the steroids, resulting in her being quite low and very tired. So it is all again a bit of a struggle. She's had to come home from school one day this week, as she is so tired. She is stiffer in the mornings, the stairs are challenging, and her fingers are still sore. I have to do buttons up again, and her jaw seems to be a little awkward when she is chewing. The doctor told us that she has s small chin due to the arthritis being present in her jaw.

The amazing thing is that she can still bend her knees. The entamacept has given her so much of her old life back.

Bethany does Physiotherapy 6 days out of 7 days as she has been given a day off.

Bethany is trying to catch up at school, this means she is not currently at the hydrotherapy sessions. Up until this year, she only missed games and drama. However, in year five she was missing math's.

She has now made a relationship with her support worker and having her has made such a difference to Bethany. She is much more secure and able to learn without worrying about her physical needs being met.

Hydrotherapy has been great. It is held at the local hospital, just in school time. Suzanne, the physiotherapist goes in the water with the children and as it is so warm, their joints relax. The water makes them feel lighter so they feel so much better. After doing their exercises, they have lots of fun and play games. The team is so dedicated to the children.

As I have said before the experience is very humbling. One of the therapy workers always has time for a chat. She has always tried to think of ways to help.

I miss the support and chats with the other parents. I hope that after Bethany has done her tests, we can go back for the summer. It would be lovely for children like Bethany to have access to hydrotherapy out of school time.

We are currently exploring the possibility of having a hot tub at home. The warm water should help ease up on the stiffness first thing in the morning. I would love to extend the facility to other children with special needs.

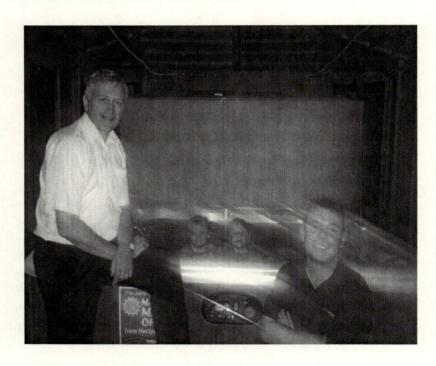

This picture shows Bethany and Mariella trying out a Hot Tub at Highway Nurseries in Norwich with John and Nathan. You can see the steam in the picture; it was a little too hot for Bethany. We would have it at the same temperature as the Hydrotherapy Pool. Hot Springs have kindly offered a discount to Bethany.

I would like to finish in thanking everyone involved in Bethany's care and especially to our families and friends. Without them, things would have been very bleak. I must drive my friends mad going on and on but they still listen.

I would like to thank the Bradwell 2nd Brownies for caring about Bethany. Snowy Owl said she had to leave the room and have a little cry during a game of musical bumps. Bethany could not get on the floor. Bethany was trying to join in even though she could not bend her legs. Snowy Owl also nominated Bethany for a Wish Come True. She was mortified that the wish went to a lady who been given a new kitchen.

Bethany has mentioned the purple evening organized by the Brownies in her story. This event has helped us all so much. By bringing Bethany's illness out into the open, she has been so much happier. Knowing how much support we have is incredible and I thank everyone who was involved in the evening. The money raised is going towards the hydrotherapy tub.

We are so lucky to be living now with science as it is, even though the drugs Bethany are taking are so new. We have to grab and enjoy all the good days.

I once said to a colleague that I wished that we could all wake up just for the day and Bethany be well. We could go to a theme park without any stress or worry. I said that I would enjoy that more than any other family there. It's so true that we don't appreciate what we have until it's gone.

Well during this journey, I have learnt not to yearn for that day anymore but to accept Bethany's limitations and as she is happy to use the wheelchair more now. We can still have good days out. We need to make this work for all of us.

The most important thing now is to encourage our children to reach their goals and aspirations even if it does take a little longer.

I hope that writing this book will really help Bethany. It's such a brave thing for her to agree to. The more she is talking to me about what to write, the more accepting she is becoming. There are feelings that I did not know she had. When she told me that she wishes she had an invisible bubble around her protecting her bumps, I felt sad but glad she is able to share it.

Bethany has helped another child by letting him watch her being injected. This will help both of them. This is a real step forward for her.

I hope that she will agree to have her photo on the front cover. I am working on that. She still does not want any attention. That is not why we are doing this. Something inside me is making me go ahead with this book.

We need to face up to our fears, as that is what paralysed us all emotionally. Fear of the unknown. We are now taking more control and pushing through the fear to free ourselves so we can all reach Bethany's little star.

Ideas to help make appointments easier

Take a notebook and another pair of ears if you can

Ask if you are not sure. Medical people can slip into their own jargon, which may not easily be understood

Ask for copies of all letters and assessments. A copy has to go to the GP so ask for your own copy. There may be points in the letter that had passed you by

Keep all copies of any letters you send to them.

Write down any questions you may have, as there is nothing worse than remembering something important when it's too late.

Try to be as specific as you can

Try to be honest about your child's suffering. Sometimes it's very difficult as a mother to describe the pain. But its very important for the professionals to get the full picture

Ask the child to say if a particular joint is sore. If your child finds it hard to talk, ask them to hold up the fingers to describe the pain if they can. Do remember that studies have shown that children play down their symptoms. You need to tell the doctor of any difficulties the child is having

If your child finds it hard to have, medical students watching them politely say no beforehand. Children really do not respond well to having many people in white coats peer over them. It is very off- putting. It is good to take someone with you. They can take your child away so that you can talk to the doctor, alone if necessary.

If you are not happy with the level of care ask your GP for a second opinion; it could help to change your child's

life.

Tips on how to keep your child's spirit up

Try to talk to your child about how he or she is feeling. If this is difficult, ask her to draw how they are feeling. Some children will find this easier and less upsetting

Keep telling your child how much they are loved and that you will always be on their side and will speak out for them when needed

Encourage everything they do, even if they can only manage a little physiotherapy due to the pain

Keep telling them over and over how proud you are of them you are. Involve them in things that they can do that make them feel less different, like swimming

Make sure your child doesn't feel somehow responsible for their illness. Explain that there are many other sick children

Bethany feels better taking control so let your child take control too. Remember they have no control over their pain

Never stop looking for new ways to help your child – never give up

Attend support groups or start one yourself

Try to find fun times for the siblings. The little research that has been done show, there are common themes between brother's and sister's. These include: low self-esteem, jealousy and guilt, academic under achievement, behavioral problems (attention seeking), anxiety and feeling left out.

Afterword

To any readers who have experienced any of this grief, pain and sorrow, my heart goes out to you, your child and all of your family.

If any words written have helped you in any small, way then all this has been worthwhile. I am delighted that the community nurses think the book will somehow change things for children.

Unless you live with a child with Arthritis, it is impossible to realize what a devastating disease it is.

It is very difficult to live in a normal way when lives are far from normal. Sometimes it feels like our lives are on hold and that we are hanging on by a thread.

Hang on, have faith. Look up for that star, it may not be out of your reach after-all.

Printed in the United Kingdom
by Lightning Source UK Ltd.
126824UK00001B/457-534/P